Diagnoses in Childhood and Adolescence for Which Pharmacotherapy May Be Therapeutically Indicated (continued)

DSM-III-R Diagnosis	Medication
Functional encopresis	(?) Lithium (p. 156)
Functional enuresis	Imipramine (p. 113)
	(?) Benzodiazepines (p. 165)
	(?) Carbamazepine (p. 176)
	(?) Amphetamines (p. 53)
	(?) Clomipramine (p. 133)
Schizophrenia	Antipsychotics (p. 78)
Mania (acute and maintenance)	Lithium (p. 151)
	Antipsychotics (p. 78)
Major depression	Antidepressants (p. 115, 120)
	(?) Lithium for prophylaxis (p. 53)
	(?) Fluoxetine (p. 139)
	(?) Clomipramine (p. 133)
Obsessive-compulsive disorder	Clomipramine (p. 131)
	(?) Fluoxetine (p. 139)
Posttraumatic stress disorder (acute)	(?) Propranolol (p. 183)
Sleep disorders	
Insomnia disorder	Benzodiazepines (p. 157)
	Diphenhydramine (p. 171)
	Hydroxyzine (p. 172)
Sleep-wake schedule disorder	Benzodiazepines (p. 157)
	Diphenhydramine (p. 171)
	Hydroxyzine (p. 172)
Sleep terror disorder	Benzodiazepines (p. 166)
	(?) Imipramine (p. 120)
	(?) Carbamazepine (p. 175)
Sleepwalking disorder	Benzodiazepines (p. 166)
	(?) Imipramine (p. 120)
Intermittent explosive disorder	(?) Propranolol (p. 181)

Child and Adolescent Clinical Psychopharmacology

Child and Adolescent Clinical Psychopharmacology

Wayne H. Green, MD

Associate Professor of Clinical Psychiatry
New York University School of Medicine
New York, New York

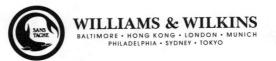

WILLIAMS & WILKINS

BALTIMORE · HONG KONG · LONDON · MUNICH
PHILADELPHIA · SYDNEY · TOKYO

Editor: Michael G. Fisher
Associate Editor: Carol Eckhart
Copy Editor: Rebecca Marnhout
Designer: Chuck Hoffman
Production Coordinator: Charles E. Zeller

Copyright © 1991
Williams & Wilkins
428 East Preston Street
Baltimore, Maryland 21202, USA

Accurate indications, adverse reactions, and dosage schedules for drugs are provided in this book, but it is possible that they may change. The reader is urged to review the package information data of the manufacturers of the medications mentioned before prescribing any medication.

Printed in the United States of America

Library of Congress Cataloging in Publication Data
Green, Wayne H.
    Child and adolescent clinical psychopharmacology / Wayne H. Green.
      p.   cm.
    Includes index.
    ISBN 0-683-03766-8
    1. Pediatric psychopharmacology.   I. Title.
    [DNLM: 1. Mental Disorders—drugs therapy. 2. Mental Disorders—in adolescence. 3. Mental Disorders—in infancy & childhood. 4. Psychopharmacology. 5. Psychotropic Drugs—therapeutic uses.   WS
350.2 G798c]
RJ504.7.G74   1991
615'.78'082—dc20
DNLM/DLC   90-13131
for Library of Congress   CIP

91 92 93 94 95
1 2 3 4 5 6 7 8 9 10

Dedicated to my parents
Albert George Green
and
Mildred Hugo Green
and my uncle and aunt
Alfred John Green
and
Ada May Green

Foreword

Psychopharmacotherapy has become a major consideration in the comprehensive psychiatric treatment of children and adolescents. Child and adolescent psychiatrists need a comprehensive, reliable text that provides them with the scientific basis and clinical methods required for applying rational, sensitive, and safe approaches to the use of psychotropic medication in children and adolescents. This book provides exactly what is needed.

Dr. Wayne Green is a master of the subject and provides the reader with a well-organized, clearly written, up-to-date account of the rationale for and the practical use of drugs. Dr. Green understands not only the multiple causes of psychiatric disorders in children and adolescents but also the multiple treatments that are needed for any given condition and, especially, the developmental factors that must be kept in mind.

This book is eminently practical. Dr. Green is clearly a seasoned clinician who puts his sound scientific knowledge and immense clinical experience in the service of other clinicians who treat troubled children and adolescents, sometimes on an urgent basis.

Dr. Green eschews a simplistic "cookbook" approach; this book is not a recipe. On the contrary, Dr. Green provides an intelligent, thoughtful, methodical, and systematic account, starting with the principles of psychopharmacotherapy and the factors to be weighed in making the many clinical decisions involved. Medicolegal responsibilities, documentation, and the complete process of administering medication from the initial dose through the termination of medication are all carefully described. Each class of drug and indications for each specific medication are carefully reviewed and considered.

One has the conviction that a clinician who reads and rereads this book, who refers to it frequently, and who follows its principles and recommendations will be on very firm ground. One might go so far as to say that no clinician should prescribe psychotropic medication for children and adolescents without having read such a book. Indeed, I can think of no other book that meets the needs of clinicians as well as does this one. Dr. Green has performed on outstanding service for the field of child and adolescent psychiatry.

Melvin Lewis, MBBS, FRC Psych, DCH
Yale Child Study Center
New Haven, Connecticut

Preface

This book is written with the conviction that proper psychiatric treatment of children and adolescents will, on some occasions, necessitate the use of psychopharmacotherapy. It is not intended to suggest that psychopharmacotherapy is warranted for most patients in this age group.

Most children and adolescents seen in private practices and in mental hygiene clinics do not require medication. Indeed, medication is not appropriate for many patients of this age group seen on inpatient psychiatric services.

Clinicians who administer psychoactive medication to children and adolescents will almost certainly encounter individuals with strong viewpoints on this treatment. Some are convinced that drugs are the answer to a child's or adolescent's problem. Others are equally certain that drugs are an anathema and ought to be avoided at all costs.

In this second, antidrug group, two lines of reasoning seem to appear with regularity in a significant minority of cases.

Some health and educational professionals working with children and adolescents maintain that in the face of compelling psychological explanations for a mental disorder, or for significant contributions to it, drugs should not be used. This group argues that drugs may have inimical effects and, further, that psychotherapy alone should be able to do the job.

A few professionals, but more often parents and relatives, offer a variation on this theme. They believe drugs should be avoided because they will make their children "zombies" or "dope them up" or "make them become drug addicts later on."

The author's point of view is that the etiology of virtually all psychiatric disorders is multiply determined. Each individual case must be fully assessed and evaluated for the potential benefits and risks of administering a specific medication. In those cases where potential benefits appear to significantly outweigh risks, usually a trial of medication is indicated.

Still, extreme caution is required in employing psychoactive medications. The long-term effects of psychoactive medications on the maturation and development of children and adolescents are at best only partially known, and many of their known untoward effects are potentially harmful.

But when a mental illness is delaying or disrupting the maturation and development of a patient, effective medication may aid considerably in bringing about more normal development and socialization. The medication often will augment the patient's ability to respond to other treatment modalities as well.

The clinician must successfully negotiate among these conflicting viewpoints and objectives in order to undertake a clinical trial of a psychoactive drug in a reasonably favorable or at least dispassionately neutral atmosphere.

Time and reality are two extremely important factors often overlooked by critics of psychopharmacotherapy. In deciding about medication, it is essential to employ a realizable goal, not some unattainable ideal.

For example, a latency-age child is diagnosed with a conduct disorder and attention deficit hyperactivity disorder. School officials threaten to suspend the child, with eventual placement in a special education class for children with behavioral problems.

In many such cases, an argument can be made that the child's problems are primarily psychological, that they could be helped by tutoring and individual and family therapies, and that medication should be withheld.

However, the realities of the case and the time frame for behavior change may call for trying medication. It may be exceedingly difficult to engage and work with the parents and the child. The child's symptoms may not have responded to the initial evaluation and intervention. The attitude of the school officials may be that the child's behavior must improve quickly.

In a situation such as this, if psychopharmacotherapy is likely to significantly hasten the therapeutic response to other treatments, or to prevent the patient from being removed from the regular classroom, the author recommends a trial of medication, unless other compelling factors are involved.

This book provides a framework for making an informed decision to undertake a clinical trial of a psychoactive medication and guides the clinician through the myriad issues involved in that decision.

Wayne H. Green, MD

Contents

Foreword *by Melvin Lewis*   vii
Preface   ix
Tables   xxiii
Figures   xxiii

Section I: Introduction and General Principles of Psychopharmacology with Children and Adolescents

1/ Introduction   3
    Overview of Book   3

2/ General Principles of Psychopharmacotherapy with Children and Adolescents   7
    Psychiatric Diagnosis and Psychopharmacotherapy   7
    CURRENT PSYCHIATRIC DIAGNOSTIC NOMENCLATURE   7
    Diagnosis and Target Symptoms   11
    Special Aspects of Child and Adolescent Psychopharmacotherapy   12
    MATURATIONAL/DEVELOPMENTAL ISSUES   12
    Physiological Factors   12
    Cognitive/Psychological/Experiential Factors   14
    RELATIONSHIP TO THE PATIENT'S FAMILY OR CARETAKERS   15
    Diagnosis, Formulation, and Development of the Treatment Plan   15
    Compliance   17
    EXPLAINING MEDICATION TO THE CHILD OR ADOLESCENT   19
    MEDICOLEGAL ASPECTS OF MEDICATING CHILDREN AND ADOLESCENTS   20

*Issues Concerning Diagnosis and Implications for
Drug Choice and Premedication Work-up*   21

Issues Concerning Informed Consent   22

Issues Concerning the Administration of Medication   23

Deviating from a Manufacturer's Labeling of a Drug   24

*Issues Concerning Documenting Ongoing
Appropriate Attention to Medication and Related
Matters in the Clinical Record*   24

Baseline Assessments Prior to Initiation of Medication   25

PHYSICAL EXAMINATION   26

LABORATORY TESTS AND DIAGNOSTIC PROCEDURES   26

Thyroid Function Tests   27

Kidney Function Tests   27

SPECIAL TESTS   27

Electrocardiogram   27

Electroencephalogram   28

BASELINE BEHAVIORAL ASSESSMENT   28

Clinical Observations   28

Rating Scales   29

Medicating the Patient   33

SELECTING THE INITIAL MEDICATION   33

Generic versus Trade Preparations   33

Standard and Nonstandard Treatments   39

DRUG INTERACTIONS   39

REGULATING THE MEDICATION   40

Selecting the Initial Dosage   40

Timing of Drug Administration   41

Scheduling Dosages   41

Drug Holidays   42

Dosage Increases   43

Titration of Medication   44

Determining the Optimal Dose   44

UNTOWARD EFFECTS (SIDE EFFECTS)   45

MONITORING OF SERUM LEVELS OF DRUGS AND/OR
THEIR METABOLITES   46

LENGTH OF TIME TO CONTINUE MEDICATION   48
Periodic Withdrawal/Tapering of Medication   49
Withdrawal Syndromes/Untoward Effects   49

Section II: Specific Drug Treatments

Introduction   53
Placebos   54
Evaluating Research Studies   56
Specific Drug Treatments   57

3/ Sympathomimetic Amines and Central Nervous System Stimulants   61
Introduction   61
Pharmacokinetics of Stimulants   63
Contraindications for Stimulant Administration   63
Interactions of Stimulants with Other Drugs   65
Untoward Effects of Stimulants   65
REBOUND EFFECTS OF STIMULANTS   66
Stimulants' Relationship to Tics and Tourette's Disorder   67
The Stimulant Drugs Approved for Use in Child and Adolescent Psychiatry   69
METHYLPHENIDATE (RITALIN)   69
Pharmacokinetics of Methylphenidate   69
Untoward Effects and Adjustment of Methylphenidate Dose Schedule   70
Investigational Reports of Interest   72
DEXTROAMPHETAMINE SULFATE (DEXEDRINE)   73
Dextroamphetamine in the Treatment of ADDH/ADHD   74
Investigational Report of Interest   74
MAGNESIUM PEMOLINE (CYLERT)   75

Magnesium Pemoline in the Treatment of ADHD   75
FENFLURAMINE (PONDIMIN)   76
Investigational Reports of Interest   77
CAFFEINE   77

4 / Antipsychotic Drugs   78
Introduction   78
Pharmacokinetics of Antipsychotics   80
Contraindications for Antipsychotic Administration   81
Interactions of Antipsychotics with Other Drugs   81
Untoward Effects of Antipsychotics   82
AGRANULOCYTOSIS   82
UNTOWARD COGNITIVE EFFECTS   82
EXTRAPYRAMIDAL SYNDROMES   82
Effects Usually Appearing during Drug Administration   83
Acute Dystonic Reactions   83
Parkinsonism (Pseudoparkinsonism)   83
Akathisia (Motor Restlessness)   84
The Prophylactic Use of Antiparkinsonian Agents for Acute Dystonic Reaction, Parkinsonism, and Akathisia   85
Neuroleptic Malignant Syndrome   87
Late-Appearing Syndromes (after Months or Years of Treatment)   87
Tardive Dyskinesia   87
Rabbit Syndrome (Perioral Tremor)   90
Other Untoward Effects of Antipsychotics   90
Representative Antipsychotics Used in Child and Adolescent Psychiatry   90
CHLORPROMAZINE (THORAZINE)   92
THIORIDAZINE (MELLARIL)   93
TRIFLUOPERAZINE (STELAZINE)   96
HALOPERIDOL (HALDOL)   96
Pharmacokinetics of Haloperidol   97
Haloperidol in the Treatment of Autistic Disorder   98

Haloperidol in the Treatment of Childhood-Onset and Atypical Pervasive Developmental Disorders   98
Haloperidol in the Treatment of Aggressive Conduct Disorder   99
THIOTHIXENE (NAVANE)   99
Investigational Report of Interest   99
CHLORPROTHIXENE (TARACTAN)   100
LOXAPINE SUCCINATE (LOXITANE)   100
Investigational Report of Interest   101
FLUPHENAZINE HYDROCHLORIDE (PROLIXIN, PERMITIL)   101
Investigational Report of Interest   102
PIMOZIDE (ORAP)   102
Pharmacokinetics of Pimozide   103
Untoward Effects of Pimozide   103
Contraindications for Pimozide Administration   103
Use of Pimozide in Children and Adolescents with Treatment-Resistant Tourette's Disorder   103
Investigational Reports of Interest   104
CLOZAPINE (CLOZARIL)   105
Untoward Effects of Clozapine   105
Investigational Report of Interest   106

5/ Antidepressants   108
Introduction   108
Tricyclic Antidepressants   108
PHARMACOKINETICS OF TRICYCLIC ANTIDEPRESSANTS   109
WITHDRAWAL OF MEDICATION   109
CONTRAINDICATIONS FOR TRICYCLIC ANTIDEPRESSANT ADMINISTRATION   110
INTERACTIONS OF TRICYCLIC ANTIDEPRESSANTS WITH OTHER DRUGS   111
UNTOWARD EFFECTS OF TRICYCLIC ANTIDEPRESSANTS   111
Tricyclic Antidepressants in Child and Adolescent Psychiatry   112
IMIPRAMINE HYDROCHLORIDE (TOFRANIL), IMIPRAMINE PAMOATE (TOFRANIL-PM)   112

Untoward Effects of Imipramine   113
Imipramine in the Treatment of Enuresis   113
Investigational Reports of Interest   115
Imipramine in the Treatment of Childhood (Prepubertal)
   Major Depressive Disorder   115
Imipramine in the Treatment of Adolescent Major Depressive
   Disorder   117
Imipramine in the Treatment of Attention Deficit Hyperactivity
   Disorder   118
Imipramine in the Treatment of Separation Anxiety Disorder
   (School Phobia)   119
Imipramine in the Treatment of Somnambulism and Night
   Terrors   120
NORTRIPTYLINE HYDROCHLORIDE (PAMELOR)   120
Investigational Reports of Interest   120
Nortriptyline in the Treatment of Major Depressive Disorder
   in Children and Adolescents   120
Nortriptyline in the Treatment of Depressed Children   121
Nortriptyline in the Treatment of Depressed Adolescents   122
*Nortriptyline Dosage Schedule for Children and
   Adolescents*   123
AMITRIPTYLINE HYDROCHLORIDE (ELAVIL, ENDEP)   125
Investigational Reports of Interest   125
Amitriptyline in Children   125
Amitriptyline in Adolescents   125
**DESIPRAMINE HYDROCHLORIDE (NORPRAMINE,
   PERTOFRANE)**   126
Investigational Reports of Interest   126
Desipramine in the Treatment of Enuresis   126
Desipramine in the Treatment of ADHD   126
Desipramine in the Treatment of Coexisting ADHD and Tics   128
CLOMIPRAMINE HYDROCHLORIDE (ANAFRANIL)   129
Pharmacokinetics of Clomipramine   130
Untoward Effects of Clomipramine   131
Investigational Reports of Interest   131

Clomipramine in the Treatment of Obsessive-Compulsive
Disorder in Children and Adolescents   131
Clomipramine in the Treatment of Attention Deficit
Hyperactivity Disorder   132
Clomipramine in the Treatment of Enuresis   133
Clomipramine in the Treatment of Depressive Symptoms   133
Clomipramine in the Treatment of School Phobia (Separation
Anxiety)   134

Monoamine Oxidase Inhibitors   134
SPECIAL CONSIDERATIONS IN USING MAOIS   135
CONTRAINDICATIONS FOR MAOI ADMINISTRATION   135
INTERACTIONS OF MAOIS WITH OTHER DRUGS   135
UNTOWARD EFFECTS OF MAOIS   136
INVESTIGATIONAL REPORTS OF INTEREST   136
MAOIs in the Treatment of Adolescent Depression   136
MAOIs in the Treatment of ADHD   136
FLUOXETINE HYDROCHLORIDE (PROZAC)   137
Pharmacokinetics of Fluoxetine   138
Contraindications for Fluoxetine Administration   138
Interactions of Fluoxetine with Other Drugs   138
Untoward Effects of Fluoxetine   138
Investigational Reports of Interest   139
Fluoxetine in the Treatment of Child and Adolescent Major
Depressive Disorders   139
Fluoxetine in the Treatment of Children and Adolescents
with Obsessive-Compulsive Disorder or Obsessive-
Compulsive Disorder and Tourette's Disorder   139

Bupropion Hydrochloride (Wellbutrin)   140
CONTRAINDICATIONS FOR BUPROPION HYDROCHLORIDE
ADMINISTRATION   140
INTERACTIONS OF BUPROPION HYDROCHLORIDE WITH
OTHER DRUGS   140
UNTOWARD EFFECTS OF BUPROPION HYDROCHLORIDE   141
INVESTIGATIONAL REPORTS OF INTEREST   141
Bupropion Hydrochloride in the Treatment of ADHD   141

6 / Lithium Carbonate   143

Introduction   143
Pharmacokinetics of Lithium Carbonate   143
Contraindications for Lithium Carbonate
  Administration   144
Interactions of Lithium Carbonate with
  Other Drugs   144
Lithium Toxicity   145
Untoward Effects of Lithium Carbonate   147
Premedication Work-up and Periodic
  Monitoring for Lithium Treatment   149
ROUTINE LABORATORY TESTS   149
Complete Blood Count with Differential   149
Serum Electrolytes   149
Pregnancy Test   149
Renal Function Tests   149
Thyroid Function Tests   150
Cardiovascular Function Tests   150
Calcium Metabolism Tests   150
Electroencephalogram   151
PERIODIC MONITORING   151
LITHIUM CARBONATE (ESKALITH, LITHANE, LITHOBID),
  LITHIUM CITRATE SYRUP (CIBALITH-S)   151
Titration of Lithium Dosage   152
The Use of Lithium Carbonate in Children under 12
  Years of Age   153
Investigational Reports of Interest   154
Lithium Carbonate in the Treatment of Mood Disorders
  (Mania, Bipolar Disorder), Behavioral Disorders with Mood
  Swings, and/or Patients Whose Parent(s) Are Lithium
  Responders   154
Lithium Carbonate in the Treatment of Disorders with Severe
  Aggression, Especially When Accompanied by Explosive
  Affect, Including Self-Injurious Behavior   155
Lithium Carbonate in the Treatment of Attention Deficit
  Hyperactivity Disorder   156

7/ Anxiolytics 157
Benzodiazepines 157
CONTRAINDICATIONS FOR BENZODIAZEPINE
   ADMINISTRATION 160
INTERACTIONS OF BENZODIAZEPINES WITH OTHER
   DRUGS 160
UNTOWARD EFFECTS OF BENZODIAZEPINES 161
USE OF BENZODIAZEPINES IN CHILD AND ADOLESCENT
   PSYCHIATRY 161
CHLORDIAZEPOXIDE (LIBRIUM) 162
Investigational Reports of Interest 162
Chlordiazepoxide in the Treatment of Behaviorally
   Disordered Children and Adolescents with Various
   Diagnoses 162
DIAZEPAM (VALIUM) 164
Investigational Reports of Interest 164
Diazepam in the Treatment of Children and Adolescents with
   Various Psychiatric Diagnoses 164
Diazepam in the Treatment of Enuresis 165
Diazepam in the Treatment of Sleep
   Disorders 166
ALPRAZOLAM (XANAX) 166
Investigational Reports of Interest 166
Azaspirodecanediones 167
BUSPIRONE HYDROCHLORIDE (BUSPAR) 167
Pharmacokinetics of Buspirone Hydrochloride 168
*Contraindications for Buspirone Hydrochloride
   Administration* 168
*Interactions of Buspirone Hydrochloride with Other
   Drugs* 168
Untoward Effects of Buspirone Hydrochloride 169
Investigational Reports of Interest 169
Buspirone Hydrochloride in the Treatment of Autistic
   Disorder 169
Buspirone Hydrochloride in the Treatment of Overanxious
   Disorder with School Phobia 169

8/ Other Drugs — 170

Antihistamines — 170

CONTRAINDICATIONS FOR ANTIHISTAMINE ADMINISTRATION — 170

INTERACTIONS OF ANTIHISTAMINES WITH OTHER DRUGS — 170

DIPHENHYDRAMINE (BENADRYL) — 171

Untoward Effects of Diphenhydramine — 172

HYDROXYZINE HYDROCHLORIDE (ATARAX), HYDROXYZINE PAMOATE (VISTARIL) — 172

Use in Child and Adolescent Psychiatry — 172

Untoward Effects of Hydroxyzine — 173

Antiepileptic Drugs — 173

CARBAMAZEPINE (TEGRETOL) — 173

Contraindications for Carbamazepine Administration — 174

Interactions of Carbamazepine with Other Drugs — 174

Investigational Reports of Interest — 174

PHENYTOIN, DIPHENYLHYDANTOIN (DILANTIN) — 177

Contraindications for Phenytoin Administration — 177

Interactions of Phenytoin with Other Drugs — 177

Use of Phenytoin in Child and Adolescent Psychiatry — 177

Opiate Antagonists — 178

NALTREXONE (TREXAN) — 178

Contraindications for Naltrexone Administration — 179

Interactions of Naltrexone with Other Drugs — 179

Use of Naltrexone in Child and Adolescent Psychiatry — 179

β-Adrenergic Blockers — 180

PROPRANOLOL (INDERAL) — 180

Contraindications for Propranolol Administration — 181

Interactions of Propranolol with Other Drugs — 181

Untoward Effects of Propranolol — 181

Use of Propranolol in Child and Adolescent Psychiatry — 181

Propranolol in the Treatment of Children and Adolescents with Brain Dysfunction, Uncontrolled Rage Outbursts, and/or Aggressiveness — 181

α-Adrenergic Antagonists   183

CLONIDINE HYDROCHLORIDE (CATAPRES), CLONIDINE
   (CATAPRES-TRANSDERMAL THERAPEUTIC SYSTEM)   183
Pharmacokinetics of Clonidine   184
Contraindications for Clonidine Administration   184
Interactions of Clonidine with Other Drugs   184
Discontinuing Medications   185
Investigational Reports of Interest   185
Clonidine in the Treatment of Attention Deficit Hyperactivity
   Disorder   185
Clonidine in the Treatment of Tourette's Disorder   188

Barbiturates and Hypnotics   189

References   190
Index   215

List of Tables and Figures

Tables

Table II.1: Diagnoses in Childhood and Adolescence for Which Pharmacotherapy May Be Therapeutically Indicated, pp. 59–60

Table 3.1: Some Pharmacokinetic Properties of Stimulant Drugs, p. 64

Table 4.1: Untoward Effects of Chlorpromazine, p. 91

Table 4.2: Antipsychotic Drugs
(Adapted from American Medical Association. Drug Evaluations. Chicago: American Medical Association, 1990.), pp. 95–96

Table 5.1: Evolution of Central Nervous System Tricyclic Toxicity
(From Preskorn SH, Jerkovick GS, Beber JH, et al., 1989), p. 110

Table 5.2: Suggested Nortriptyline Dose Schedules for Children and Adolescents
(From Geller B, Cooper TB, Chestnut EC, et al., 1985), p. 124

Table 6.1: Lithium Carbonate Dosage Guide for Prepubertal School-Age Children
(From Weller EB, Weller RA, Fristad MA, 1986.), p. 154

Table 7.1: Some Representative Benzodiazepines, p. 162

Figures

Figure 1: Conners Parent-Teacher Questionnaire
(Modified, from Department of Health, Education, and Welfare, Health Services and Mental Health Administration, National Institute of Mental Health), pp. 30–31

Figure 2: Abnormal Involuntary Movement Scale (AIMS)
(Modified, from Department of Health, Education, and Welfare, Public Health Services, Alcohol, Drug Abuse, and Mental Health Administration, National Institute of Mental Health), pp. 34–37

Section I

Introduction and General Principles of Psychopharmacology with Children and Adolescents

1

Introduction

OVERVIEW OF BOOK

This book will review selected topics and representative drugs used in child and adolescent psychopharmacology from a practical, clinically oriented perspective and is intended primarily for clinicians actively engaged in treating children and adolescents with psychoactive medication. This includes child psychiatrists, residents in general psychiatry who are treating children and adolescents, residents specializing in child and adolescent psychiatry, pediatric residents, and other physicians who may prescribe drugs to patients in this age range. In addition, other clinicians and mental health personnel who work with children who are receiving psychoactive medication may wish to review the medications their patients are receiving.

The first part of the book focuses rather intensively on the general principles of psychopharmacotherapy with children and adolescents. The reader is presented with a clinically useful way of thinking about psychopharmacotherapy, beginning with the initial clinical contact and continuing through the psychiatric evaluation, psychodynamic formulation, diagnosis, and development of the treatment plan. For those cases where psychoactive medication is advocated as a part of the treatment plan, the necessary medicolegal responsibilities of the clinician in introducing and explaining the purpose of medication to the patient and relevant caretakers, ways of maximizing the chances of the patient's and his or her legal guardians' accepting a trial of the medication and their cooperating with its administration, and the necessary documentation of these facts in the clinical record are reviewed. Following this, the entire process of administering medication is discussed. This begins with consideration of which drug to choose for the initial trial of medication, the necessary documentation of target symptoms and any baseline behavioral ratings that will be useful in assessing clinical response or the development of untoward effects, and which baseline physical and laboratory assessments to select.

This first part of the book ends with a detailed presentation of the principles of administering psychoactive medication from the initial dose, through titration and determining the optimal dose, to maintenance therapy, duration of treatment, and issues in terminating medication. These principles are generalizable and provide clinical guidelines for selecting and administering any psychoactive medication to children and adolescents.

The second portion of the book begins with a brief discussion of the history of child psychopharmacology and some issues concerning psychopharmacological research in children and adolescents. The purpose of this is to remind the reader of where the information that follows is placed in the history of child psychopharmacology and of the importance of research and a critical assessment of the presented data for informed clinical practice.

After these brief introductory comments, the remainder of Part II of the book focuses on specific psychopharmacological agents that are presently the most important in the clinical practice of child and adolescent psychiatry. These drugs are presented by class. Many specific psychoactive medications are presently used to treat diverse psychiatric disorders or symptoms across psychiatric diagnoses (e.g., lithium's use for its antiaggressive effects), and this method of organization avoids repeating similar information under several diagnoses. Equally important, as we learn more about the etiopathogenesis of psychiatric disorders, it becomes increasingly useful, both scientifically and clinically, to think about how drugs affect basic neurotransmitter and psychoneuroendocrine functioning across diagnoses. A given drug may affect one or more neurotransmitter systems. Likewise, a specific neurotransmitter system may be important in one or more diagnostic categories. For example, there appears to be a relationship between the serotonergic system's functioning and aggressive or violent behavior and self-destructive behavior among various diagnostic groups (Linnoila et al., 1989; Mann et al., 1989). (Recently an entire book devoted solely to the behavioral pharmacology of serotonin was published [Bevan et al., 1989]).

As might be expected in a clinically oriented book, the standard psychopharmacological treatments established by investigational and clinical studies as both efficacious and safe for use in children and adolescents and approved by the Federal Drug Administration (FDA) for advertising as such are emphasized. The literature reviews determining the efficacy of these treatments, however, are kept to a minimum, as comprehensive reviews are readily available elsewhere. (For the interested reader a list of such additional readings is given in the introductory comments to Part II of this book.)

The author emphasizes that no book can substitute for a careful reading of the manufacturer's labeling, which is packaged with drugs and is reprinted verbatim in the current *Physicians' Desk Reference* (PDR) and its supplements, unless, of course, the book itself reprints verbatim the package insert. The FDA-approved labeling (package insert) contains additional information on all FDA-approved medications discussed in this book. No drug should be prescribed without the physician's having read and become familiar with its labeling information; to do so is a disservice to one's patient and renders one vulnerable to professional liability.

In addition to standard treatments, however, selected medications currently prescribed to children and adolescents for unlabeled (non-FDA-approved) indications and medications that have recently been under clinical investigation and with which the clinician should be familiar are reviewed. (In a very few cases investigational drugs not yet approved by the FDA for any use are discussed. Such drugs are usually available only through research protocols; in some cases they may be available in other countries. Typically these drugs are not used in ordinary clinical practice.) Medications that appear to be possible candidates for eventual approval as standard treatments (e.g., clomipramine, which was recently approved by the FDA for treating symptoms of obsessive-compulsive disorder in persons at least 10 years of age but is still not approved for younger children) or that may be clinically important when patients do not respond to standard treatments are emphasized. Because reviews of these medications are usually less readily available and some studies are very recent, relevant studies are summarized herein. Although this relative emphasis on the literature of studies of drugs used for non-FDA-approved or unlabeled indications over FDA-approved drugs may seem paradoxical, it is deliberate. This is because, in clinical practice, a major difficulty occurs when a patient does not respond with sufficient amelioration of symptoms to standard pharmacological treatments currently available. When, despite treatment with standard medications, the patient's symptoms prevent him or her from functioning in a psychosocial environment that will facilitate normal growth, maturation, and development, many clinicians will consider the possibility of using FDA-approved drugs for non-FDA-approved indications to treat their patient. While not proselytizing for the use of medication for non-FDA-approved uses, this book does present the clinician with possible alternative treatments for patients who are resistant to standard pharmacological treatments. In fact, the use of some of these medications for nonlabeled indications is medically accepted in clinical practice.

As with standard treatments, the physician must consider, perhaps even more carefully, the risks versus the potential benefits of using any medication for non-FDA-approved indications. Medicolegal and some practical issues of using nonstandard treatments are considered below in the appropriate sections of the book.

General Principles of Psychopharmacotherapy with Children and Adolescents

PSYCHIATRIC DIAGNOSIS AND PSYCHOPHARMACOTHERAPY

Psychopharmacotherapy should always be part of a comprehensive treatment plan arrived at after a thorough psychiatric evaluation that results in a diagnosis, or at minimum a working diagnosis. It is scientifically indefensible to initiate treatment without first attempting to formulate as clear an understanding of the clinical picture as possible. This will enable the clinician to institute the most appropriate and rational treatment(s) available in his or her therapeutic armamentarium for the situation at hand.

Current Psychiatric Diagnostic Nomenclature

A major difficulty with the official American Psychiatric Association (APA) nomenclature, the *Diagnostic and Statistical Manual of Mental Disorders, Third Edition, Revised* (DSM-III-R) (APA, 1987), and indeed with most current psychiatric nomenclatures is that usually etiology is not taken into account in formulating a diagnosis. One reason for this is that, at our present state of knowledge, we do not know the etiologies of many conditions. Hence we are often treating specific constellations of behavioral

7

symptoms without understanding adequately their biological and genetic underpinnings and how they interact with their psychosocial and physical environments. For example, autistic disorder is not etiologically homogeneous but has a multitude of causes.

Theoretically, drugs may be effective for a given psychiatric disorder by correcting the condition(s) leading to it or by influencing events somewhere along the usually complex pathways between the hypothesized abnormality(-ies) and its subsequent psychological and/or behavioral consequences. Thus some psychoactive drugs may be effective in several dissimilar disorders because they influence or modify neurotransmitters and psychoneuroendocrine events in the brain along or near the end of these interacting, partially confluent, or final common pathways. Other psychoactive drugs appear to exert their therapeutic effects through entirely different mechanisms in different diagnostic entities; for example, imipramine in depression, attention deficit hyperactivity disorder (ADHD), and enuresis.

Some patients with a specific diagnosis (e.g., ADHD, autistic disorder, or schizophrenia) will not have a satisfactory clinical response or will be refractory to a specific drug—even one known to be highly effective in statistically significant double-blind studies—or will even have a worsening of symptoms. This may reflect differences in genetic makeup or other biologically determined conditions, psychosocial environments, and/or internalized conflicts and the contributions each makes to the etiopathogenesis of each patient's psychiatric disorder.

While diagnostic issues are not specifically treated in this book, it is emphasized that an accurate diagnosis may be of critical importance in choosing the correct medication. For example, Bowden and Sarabia (1980), Carlson and Strober (1978), and Horowitz (1977) reported on a total of 17 adolescents with bipolar manic-depressive disorder who were initially misdiagnosed as having schizophrenia. Most of the patients with bipolar disorder who were diagnosed incorrectly were treated with antipsychotics and failed to show clinical improvement or responded poorly. When subsequently correctly rediagnosed with manic-depressive disorder and treated with lithium carbonate, the patients showed remarkable improvements or complete remissions of their psychoses. Horowitz (1977) noted that the presence of mood disturbance with marked lability and prominent elevations and depressions, grandiosity and flight of ideas, and pressured speech, hyperactivity, and distractibility predicted lithium-responsive manic-depression (bipolar disorder) even when massive alterations of thinking and hallucinations were present. Thus at times the lack of expected clinical response to a medication should suggest to the clinician the possibility of an incorrect diagnosis and that a careful diagnostic reconsideration should be undertaken.

Other unfortunate clinical consequences may result from incorrect diagnoses. For example, antidepressants may precipitate an acute psychotic reaction when given to individuals with schizophrenic disorder. Stimulant medications, too, may precipitate psychosis when given to children or adolescents with borderline personalities or unrecognized schizophrenia.

Wender (1988) noted that clinical experience suggested that some children diagnosed with ADHD who were treated with stimulants and rapidly developed tolerance to them were actually suffering from a major depressive disorder and that they responded to treatment with tricyclic antidepressants with remarkable improvement.

Changing diagnostic criteria may also complicate matters. For example, some of the controversy regarding the efficacy of stimulants in the mentally retarded may have resulted from diagnostic issues. Until the publication of the *Diagnostic and Statistical Manual of Mental Disorders, Second Edition* (DSM-II) by the APA in 1968, there was no specific APA diagnosis for what was commonly known as the hyperactive child. There were various labels for this condition including hyperactive child, hyperkinetic syndrome, minimal brain dysfunction, and minimal cerebral dysfunction. One influential definition of minimal brain dysfunction was that of the Minimal Brain Dysfunction National Project on Learning Disabilities in Children in 1966. This report defined minimal brain dysfunction (MBD) to designate

> children of near average, average, or above average general intelligence with certain learning and/or behavioral disabilities ranging from mild to severe, which are associated with deviations of function of the central nervous system. These deviations may manifest themselves by various combinations of impairment in perception, conceptualization, language, memory, and control of attention, impulse, or motor function. These aberrations may arise from genetic variations, biochemical irregularities, perinatal insults or other illnesses or injuries sustained during the years which are critical for the development and maturation of the central nervous system, or from other unknown organic causes. (Clements, 1966, p. 53)

Mental retardation was considered evidence of more than "minimal" dysfunction, and the various etiologies were felt to be biological. Because of this concept, children with mental retardation were excluded from the possibility of receiving a codiagnosis of minimal brain dysfunction, hyperactive child, or an equivalent diagnosis, and some clinicians may not have tried stimulant medication in their patients who had even mild mental retardation.

The situation changed with the publication of DSM-II, which noted that "in children, mild brain damage often manifests itself by hyperactivity, short attention span, easy distractibility, and impulsiveness" (APA, 1968, p. 31) and suggested that unless there are significant interactional factors (e.g., between child and parents) that appear to be responsible for these behaviors, the disorder should be classified as a nonpsychotic organic brain syndrome and not as a behavior disorder such as hyperkinetic reaction of childhood or adolescence. DSM-II conceptualized hyperkinetic reaction of childhood as a reactive disorder secondary to internalization of interpersonal conflicts with resulting characteristic symptoms. There was no other available category for a child or adolescent of normal intelligence who exhibited such symptoms as his or her natural baseline of behavior, unless one assumed some degree of brain damage.

In DSM-III (APA, 1980a), the diagnosis of attention deficit disorder with hyperactivity (ADDH) was based on the presence of a specific constellation of symptoms and no etiology was hypothesized. Hence children of any intelligence could exhibit such features. DSM-III additionally notes that mild or moderate mental retardation may predispose to the development of ADDH and that the addition of this diagnosis to the severely and profoundly retarded is not clinically useful as these symptoms are often an inherent part of the condition.

DSM-III-R redefines ADDH somewhat, renames it attention-deficit hyperactivity disorder (ADHD), and refines its relationship to mental retardation. It notes that many features of ADHD may be present in mentally retarded persons because of the generalized delays in intellectual development. A mentally retarded child or adolescent should be additionally diagnosed with ADHD only if the relevant symptoms significantly exceed those that are compatible with the child's or adolescent's mental age.

DIAGNOSIS AND TARGET SYMPTOMS

In making the decision as to which psychoactive medication to select initially, two major issues should be addressed: diagnosis and target symptoms. Both are important and are often interrelated. It is essential to make an accurate diagnosis and to identify and quantify target symptoms in order to choose an efficacious drug and to assess the results of medication. The target symptoms must be of sufficient severity and must interfere so significantly with the child's or adolescent's current functioning and future maturation and development that the potential benefits of the drug will justify the risks concomitant with its administration.

The initial medication may be chosen with respect to either diagnosis or target symptoms or both. Sometimes the decision is not difficult, as the same medication is appropriate for both the target symptoms and the diagnosis. For example, antipsychotics are the drugs of first choice for treating schizophrenia and are also appropriate for most of the significant target symptoms (e.g., hallucinations, thought disorder, and delusions).

The symptom "hyperactivity," however, is present in numerous childhood psychiatric disorders, but all hyperactivity is not the same. The clinician should be fully aware of the diagnosis in treating this symptom. Hyperactivity in a youngster with ADHD would be expected to respond favorably to the administration of a stimulant, while a schizophrenic youngster who is in relative remission but exhibits marked hyperactivity would have a good chance of having his or her psychotic symptoms reexacerbated were stimulant medication used. Stimulant drugs, the drugs of choice in ADHD, are considered to be relatively contraindicated in schizophrenia and may cause worsening of psychotic symptoms.

Medication also can be prescribed to treat certain specific diagnoses. Lithium, for example, has a certain specificity for treatment of mania in patients diagnosed with bipolar disorder, manic, but also appears to have an antiaggressive action that cuts across various diagnoses. Lithium has been used effectively to treat aggression directed against others or self-injurious behavior, in children and adolescents diagnosed with conduct disorder, mental retardation with disturbance of behavior, and autistic disorder.

SPECIAL ASPECTS OF CHILD PSYCHOPHARMACOTHERAPY

Maturational/Developmental Issues

Physiological Factors

The relationship of biological developmental issues to psychopharmacotherapy has been emphasized in the recent book *Psychiatric Pharmacosciences of Children and Adolescents* (Popper, 1987b). Children and adolescents often require larger doses of psychoactive medication per unit of body weight than adults do to attain similar blood levels and therapeutic efficacy. It is usually assumed that two factors explain this: more rapid metabolism by the liver and an increased glomerular filtration rate in children compared to that in adults. The latter suggests a greater renal clearance for some drugs, including lithium, which helps to explain the fact that therapeutic dosages of lithium in children do not differ from those in adults (Campbell et al., 1984a).

Teicher and Baldessarini (1987) pointed out that children may respond to drugs differently from adults because of pharmacodynamic factors (drug-effector mechanisms) that are caused by developmental changes in neural pathways or their functions or because of pharmacokinetic factors caused by developmental changes in the distribution, metabolism, or excretion of a drug.

Jatlow (1987) has noted that although the rapid rate of drug disposition may decrease gradually throughout childhood, around puberty there may be an abrupt decline. Drug disposition usually reaches adult levels by mid- to late adolescence. Clinically, this would indicate that the clinician should be especially alert to possible changes in pharmacokinetics during the time period around puberty and be ready to adjust dose levels if necessary. When they are available, it may be useful to obtain plasma concentration levels if there appears to be a change in the clinical efficacy of a drug as a child matures into an adolescent.

Puig-Antich (1987) summarized some of the evidence that catecholamine (norepinephrine, epinephrine, and dopamine) systems are not fully anatomically developed and operationally functional until adulthood. The relatively high prevalence of ADHD in younger children and its spontaneous improvement in many children with the passage of time may reflect maturational changes in catecholamine function. Interestingly, both the fact that younger children respond to stimulant medication differently from older adolescents and adults with respect to affect or mood and do not report elation, excitation, or euphoria and the fact that mania and euphoria are relatively rare in childhood may also be explained by the immaturity of the catecholamine systems (Puig-Antich, 1987) and can be considered to result from developmental pharmacodynamic factors.

Similarly, the pharmacokinetics of many drugs change over the course of life. Children and younger adolescents many differ from older adolescents and adults, as the elderly may again differ from middle-aged persons. For example, children and adolescents under 15 years of age treated with clomipramine had significantly lower steady-state plasma concentrations for a given dose than did adults (see package insert). Rivera-Calimlim et al. (1979) reported that children and adolescents 8 to 15 years of age required larger doses of chlorpromazine than adults to attain similar plasma concentrations.

There may also be differences between acute and chronic pharmacokinetics. For example, Sallee et al. (1985) noted in one subject that magnesium pemoline elimination half-time almost doubled from 7.5 hours after an acute dose to 14.3 hours after 3 weeks of treatment with magnesium pemoline. Rivera-Calimlim et al. (1979) reported a decline in plasma chlorpromazine levels in most of their child and adolescent patients who were on a fixed dose and suggested it might be due to autoinduction of metabolic enzymes for chlorpromazine during long-term treatment, as had been reported previously in adults.

Puig-Antich noted that there was a clear relationship between plasma concentrations and clinical response to imipramine for prepubescent subjects and older subjects with endogenous depression, but not for adolescents (Burke & Puig-Antich, 1990). He hypothesized that the relatively poor clinical efficacy of tricyclic antidepressants in postpubescent adolescents and young adults compared to the clinical response of prepubescent children and older adults is secondary to increased sex hormone levels' having a negative effect on the antidepressant action of imipramine. Because of this, monoamine oxidase inhibitors may be of particular use in selected depressed adolescents who do not respond satisfactorily to tricyclic antidepressants.

Herskowitz (1987) has reviewed the developmental neurotoxicity of pharmacoactive drugs. Developmental neurotoxicity is concerned with stage-specific drug-induced biochemical or physiological changes, morphological manifestations, and behavioral symptoms. For example, stimulant medication may adversely affect normal increases in height and growth, at least temporarily, in some actively growing children and adolescents. Some psychoactive drugs taken during early pregnancy have significant potential for damaging the fetus (e.g., lithium may cause cardiac malformations).

Cognitive/Psychological/Experiential Factors

The maturation and development of the central nervous system as well as the life experiences accumulating since infancy determine much of the specific level of functioning of a given child or adolescent. Although detailed knowledge of these factors is essential in order to evaluate psychiatrically any child or adolescent, herein only their specific relevance to psychopharmacotherapy will be addressed.

In general, the younger the patient, the less verbal facility is available to convey information to the clinician and reciprocally to understand information the clinician wishes to impart. Part of the psychiatric evaluation leading to a decision that psychotropic medication is indicated will provide the clinician with an assessment of the level of the patient's ability to communicate his or her emotional status and of his or her cognitive/linguistic ability to understand the proposed treatment and reliably report how the treatment is affecting him or her.

In the very young child or the child with no communicative language, the clinician can only observe behavioral effects of medication directly or learn of them as reported by others. The younger the child, the fewer complaints (or compliments) about beneficial or untoward effects. Also, the young child has less-differentiated emotions and more limited experience with feelings and emotions and with communicating them to others than older children have. In addition, some chronically depressed or anxious children may not have had a sufficiently recent normal emotional baseline to which they can compare their present mood. Such children may experience a depressed mood as their normal, usual state of being and thus do not have a normal baseline frame of reference upon which to draw in describing how they feel.

The younger the child, the less accurate are time estimates. Until about 10 years of age, concepts of long periods of time are often not easily understood. It can be very useful and at times essential to use concrete markers of time in discussing time concepts and chronology of events with children. For example, the clinician may inquire if something occurred before or after the last birthday, specific holidays (e.g., Christmas, Thanksgiving, or Halloween), specific events, (e.g., separation or divorce of parents, when the family moved to another home, an operation, a relative's death, or the birth of a sibling), the seasons or weather (e.g., winter, snow, cold or summer, hot), or the school year (e.g., specific teacher's name or grade or Christmas, spring or Easter, or summer vacation).

Concepts such as concentration, distractibility, and impulsivity may be beyond the understanding of some early latency-age children. Different children may use different words or expressions to express the same concept. It is important to be certain a child knows the meaning of a specific word and not just assume this is the case because he or she responds to a question. If there is any doubt, ask what something means or explain it in another way. It can be very useful to ask the same thing in several different ways.

In the final analysis, once the patient's psychopathology and his or her developmental experiential factors are taken into account, it is the quality of the relationship between the clinician and the child or adolescent that becomes paramount in determining the usefulness of information shared.

Relationship to the Patient's Family or Caretakers

Diagnosis, Formulation, and Development of the Treatment Plan

A complete psychiatric assessment, including appropriate psychological tests, resulting in a working diagnosis and comprehensive treatment plan; appropriate physical and laboratory examinations; and baseline behavioral measurements should be completed as minimum prerequisites prior to the initiation of psychopharmacotherapy. The treatment plan should be developed in conjunction with both the parents or the primary caretaker and include participation of the child or adolescent as appropriate to his or her understanding. Treatment with psychoactive drugs should always be part of a more comprehensive treatment regimen and rarely, if ever, is appropriate as the sole treatment modality for a child or adolescent.

At variance with this traditional wisdom, however, are the results of several studies comparing treatment of hyperactive children with stimulant medication alone versus stimulant medication combined with other interventions, such as cognitive training, attention control, social reinforcement, and parent training. A recent review of these studies concluded that "the additional use of various forms of psychotherapies (behavioral treatment, parent training, cognitive therapy) with stimulants has not resulted in superior outcomes than medication alone" (Klein, 1987, p. 1223). One possible factor contributing to this result is that in several studies children who were treated with methylphenidate alone showed improvement in social behavior. Following this, adults, both parents and teachers, related to the children more positively (Klein, 1987). It seems clinically unlikely, however, that all the difficulties of ADHD children are secondary to the target symptoms that improve with methylphenidate. Those difficulties that result from other psychosocial difficulties, including psychopathological familial interactions and long-standing maladaptive behavioral patterns, would be expected to benefit from additional interventions, and until it is possible to differentiate those children whose difficulties arise from their attention deficit per se from children whose symptoms are of multidetermined origin, a comprehensive treatment program is recommended for all children, including those with ADHD.

The legal guardian and the child or adolescent patient, to the degree appropriate to the patient's age and psychopathology, should participate in formulating the treatment plan. The use of medication, including expected benefits and possible short- and long-term untoward effects, should be reviewed with the parents and patient in understandable terminology. Their informed consents should be obtained and included in the clinical record.

It is essential to assess carefully the attitude and reliability of the persons who will be responsible for administering the medication. Unless there is a positive or at least honestly neutral attitude toward medication and some therapeutic alliance with the parents, it will be difficult or infeasible to make a reliable assessment of drug efficacy and compliance. Likewise, to store and administer medication safely on an outpatient basis requires a responsible adult, especially if there are young children in the home or if the patient is at suicidal risk.

It should be explained to parents that even if medication helps some symptoms that are biologically determined (e.g., in some cases of ADHD), the disorder's presence may have in turn caused psychological difficulties in the child or adolescent himself or herself, as well as disturbances in familial and social relationships. Controlling or ameliorating the biological difficulty usually does not immediately correct the long-standing internalized psychological or interpersonal problems. Resolving these difficulties will take time and may often require concomitant individual, group, family, or other therapeutic modalities.

Compliance

Compliance is an issue of particular importance in child and adolescent psychiatry, and because the parents or other caretakers usually are interposed between physician and patient, it is somewhat more complex than in adult psychiatry, where the patient usually relates directly to the physician.

Obviously, for psychopharmacotherapy to be effective in the disorder for which it is prescribed, the drug must be taken following the prescribed directions. Erratic compliance or running out of medication may cause the patient to undergo what is in effect an abrupt withdrawal of medication. Withdrawal syndromes may sometimes be confused with untoward effects, worsening of the clinical condition, or inadequate medication levels. In some cases (e.g., when an antipsychotic is used) the patient is at increased risk for an acute dystonic reaction if the physician starts at the optimal dose after the drug has been discontinued for several days or more. In addition, when medication is stopped, it may sometimes require a higher dose of medication to regain the same degree of symptom control. For example, Sleator et al. (1974) found that 7 of 28 hyperactive children who showed clinical worsening during a month-long placebo period after having received methylphenidate for 1 to 2 years required an increase in dose to regain their original clinical improvement. Hence it is very important to emphasize to parents that running out of medication is to be avoided.

Many factors may interfere with compliance. Some parents will at times withhold medication if their child appears to be doing well, or, conversely, increase the medication without the physician's approval if the patient's behavior worsens, or even administer the drug to the child as a punishment.

When parents or legal guardians seek treatment for their children primarily because of pressure from others, such as a school, a child welfare agency, or a court, there may be considerable resistance to both treatment and medication. Some of these parents may delay filling the prescription, lose it, or simply not fill it. Other parents consider it something to be done when convenient, especially if they have to travel any distance to get the prescription filled. If money is involved, even a small sum to pay for the prescription or for travel, some families, especially those on public assistance or very limited budgets, may have to delay purchasing the medication for legitimate financial reasons. These issues may come into play each time the prescription is renewed; additionally, it is not rare in many clinics for parents to miss appointments, including those when medication is to be renewed.

At times, some children and adolescents, both outpatients and inpatients, may actively try to avoid ingesting medication. Their techniques include pretending to place the pill in their mouths and later discarding the pill, and placing the pill under the tongue or between teeth and the cheek when swallowing and later spitting it out. Compliance in these cases may be improved if the person administering the medication observes it in the mouth and watches the patient swallow it. Crushing the medication may be helpful in some cases, but one must be certain absorption rates will not be so significantly altered as to cause decreased clinical efficacy or untoward or toxic effects. If available, switching to a liquid form of the drug may be indicated for some patients.

Another factor that influences compliance, particularly in older children and adolescents, is related to untoward effects. For example, if they feel "funny" or different or develop a stomachache, they may be more reluctant to take medication. The more responsible a child is for administering his or her own medication, the more likely in general unpleasant, untoward effects will interfere with compliance. Akathisia is a particularly unpleasant untoward effect that Van Putten and Marder (1987) found increased the likelihood of noncompliance in adults receiving antipsychotics. Sheard (1975) has noted that individuals treated for aggressive behavior may poorly tolerate untoward effects and discontinue treatment to avoid them. It is likely these and other untoward effects would have similar effects on children and adolescents.

Noncompliance may be lessened sometimes if an adequate, understandable explanation of the simple pharmacokinetics of the drug is given to parents and patients when initially discussing medication; for example, the importance of keeping blood levels fairly constant by taking the medication as prescribed can be emphasized and reviewed again if lack of compliance becomes important. On the other hand, when parents continue to sabotage treatment either consciously, unconsciously, because of their own psychopathology, or for other reasons, and this seriously interferes with the psychiatric treatment of a child or adolescent, it may be necessary to report the patient to a governmental agency as a case of medical neglect and request legal intervention. Likewise, it may be necessary to discontinue medication if compliance is very poor or so unacceptably erratic as to be potentially dangerous.

Explaining Medication to the Child or Adolescent

The clinician should discuss the medication with the child or adolescent as appropriate to the patient's psychopathology and ability to understand. Giving the patient an opportunity to participate in his or her treatment is helpful for many reasons.

The patient can feel like an active partner in his or her treatment. This can alleviate feelings of passivity—that something over which the patient has no control is being done to him or her. Letting the patient know that he or she should pay attention to the effects of the medication in order to be able to report them to the therapist, that the patient will be listened to, and that what the patient conveys will be seriously considered in regulating the medicine also helps the therapeutic relationship. The patient also can be informed that even though medication may be able to provide some relief or help, it cannot do everything, and he or she still must contribute effort toward reaching the treatment goals. This can be particularly important during adolescence, when issues of autonomy and control over one's own body are normal developmental concerns.

As the patient is experiencing firsthand the disorder being treated, in many cases valuable information necessary for regulating the medication can be obtained directly. Some quite young children can express whether the medicine makes them feel better, more calm or quiet; less mad or less like fighting; happier or sadder; less afraid, upset, nervous, or anxious; or worse, sleepy, tired, more bored, madder, or harder to get along with other kids, and so on. Although parents or caretakers can provide much useful information, they may be unaware of some information the patient can provide if time is taken to learn the words or expressions that the child uses to communicate feelings and experiences.

Untoward effects should be explained according to the understanding and situation of the child or adolescent. The patient's awareness that untoward effects may be transient (e.g., tolerance for sedation may develop) or reversible with dose reduction may be helpful in gaining cooperation during the titration period. Foreknowledge also increases the sense of control and can decrease fear of some untoward effects. For example, if an acute dystonic reaction is a possibility, it is important to realize how frightening this can be to some patients (and their parents). Discussing beforehand that if this occurs, medicine will help and it will go away can make the experience less frightening. Also, if a rapidly effective oral anticholinergic is made available and patients and parents are aware of what is happening, the medication may be administered earlier in the process, frequently aborting a potentially more severe reaction.

Children who ride bicycles and adolescents who may drive a car, motor bike, or motorcycle or operate potentially dangerous machinery should be cautioned if a medication may cause sedation or other impairment to wait until they sure how they are reacting to the medication before engaging in these activities. Similarly, if an adolescent is likely to use alcohol or other psychoactive drugs, he or she should be warned of possible additive or other adverse effects. Drugs like monoamine oxidase inhibitors cannot be used without very cooperative patients who are able to follow necessary dietary restrictions.

Medicolegal Aspects of Medicating Children and Adolescents

Medicolegal issues usually involve concerns about the clinician's clinical competence, and although it may be obvious, these issues arise primarily when something goes wrong. Incidentally, that "wrong something" may have nothing to do with the clinician's specific treatment or competence but may be, for example, an outcome that displeases the patient or guardian. Even then, for a medicolegal issue to arise, someone who has become aware of it has to decide to pursue the matter legally.

The importance of the above is that the clinician's relationship with the patient and his or her family or caretakers can either increase or decrease the likelihood of legal action. As a general rule, the better the quality of the relationship and rapport between the physician and patient and his or her family, the less likely is legal action to occur. Parents who are angry at their child's physician, who feel neglected or not cared about, are more likely to institute legal action. Taking time to explain what the medicine may do and may not do is important; no medication can be guaranteed to be clinically effective and safe for every patient.

If there is a risk a depressed patient may make a suicide attempt but the patient is not hospitalized, this should be discussed with all concerned parties. The patient may be asked to commit verbally or in writing to a contract to contact the clinician before any attempt to take his or her own life. Legal guardians should be informed of and concur with the decision that their child or ward will not be hospitalized and that, although there is a risk, the degree of risk is acceptable to avoid hospitalization. The guardians should be asked to provide more formal supervision until the depression improves sufficiently. If such measures are carried out and documented and a working rapport established, the risk of legal action and/or liability will be lessened should a suicide attempt, successful or otherwise, occur.

The clinician should make a genuine effort to establish a working rapport with parents who have consented to the treatment of their child or adolescent under duress (e.g., because a governmental agency has placed legal pressure on them to comply with treatment), although this is frequently difficult.

Holzer (1989) noted that most if not all malpractice claims occur in cases with either an unexpected clinical outcome or an event that is perceived by the patient (or parents) as avoidable or preventable. The aspects of psychopharmacotherapy that have potential for medicolegal difficulties parallel this book's entire section on general principles of psychopharmacotherapy. Lawsuits are most frequently brought if something is omitted or if something goes wrong that could reasonably have been prevented. It should be emphasized that proper documentation in the clincial record is essential. If this is not done, the clinician's position is precarious if legal difficulties arise. Particular areas of concern are discussed below.

Issues Concerning Diagnosis and Implications for Drug Choice and Premedication Work-up

The areas of major concern here are making a correct psychiatric diagnosis and being aware of any coexisting medical conditions. Taking accurate medical and psychiatric histories, including previous medications and the patient's response to them, including untoward effects and allergic reactions, is essential. Nurcombe (1990) notes that if adverse reactions to a drug or drug interactions occur that could have been predicted by taking an accurate and adequate history, the physician may be held liable. History taking must be followed by a proper premedication work-up and, if the patient has a medical condition, consideration of how the psychotropic medication would affect that condition and of any drug interactions with other medications the patient is taking.

Some examples of this include (a) making an incorrect diagnosis and prescribing the wrong medication, or failing to detect or recognize coexisting conditions that would make the chosen medication contraindicated; (b) prescribing a drug that will interact adversely with another medication the patient is taking, or a prescribing a drug to which the patient has been previously allergic; or (c) failing to perform a baseline ECG if tricyclics are to be used for indications other than enuresis and there is a possibility of reaching cardiotoxic blood levels.

Issues Concerning Informed Consent

The treatment plan should be discussed and agreed to by the legal guardian and the patient as appropriate for his or her age and understanding. The diagnosis, risks, and benefits of the proposed treatment and alternative treatment possibilities should be reviewed. To give informed consent, a patient (or legal guardian) must be mentally competent, have sufficient information available to make an informed decision, and not be coerced. Adolescents 12 years of age and older should participate formally in developing their treatment plans and in giving informed consent. If this is not possible, it should be so stated in the clinical record. It is wise to have both the legal guardian and, when appropriate, the patient sign the treatment plan and/or an informed consent for medication. If this is not done, at a minimum the clinician must document the discussion of the treatment plan and the response of the patient and legal guardian to this in the clinical record.

Nurcombe (1990) recommends that the following be discussed:

a. The nature of the condition that requires treatment.
b. The nature and purpose of the proposed treatment and the probability that it will succeed.
c. The risks and consequences of the proposed treatment.
d. Alternatives to the proposed treatment and their attendant risks and consequences.
e. Prognosis with and without the proposed treatment (p. 1132).

Popper (1987a) adds that it should be explicitly stated that there may be unknown risks to taking the medication, especially when using novel psychopharmacological treatments or treatments where risks versus benefits are uncertain.

Involuntary medication of patients occurs primarily in emergency rooms and on inpatient wards. This is usually permissible in a true emergency, but Nurcombe (1990) cautions that even involuntary commitment to a hospital for psychiatric treatment permits involuntary medication only in narrowly defined circumstances. Administering medication forcibly without judicial approval in a nonemergency situation may be considered battery. Physicians should become thoroughly familiar with their state laws and local hospital policies governing these matters.

Issues Concerning the Administration of Medication

The issues include justification for the decision to use medication in treating the psychiatric condition (risks versus benefits), rationale for the initial drug chosen, and administering the drug by the appropriate route (orally, intramuscularly, or intravenously) and in a clinically efficacious dose. If a patient is suicidal, the prescribing physician should ascertain to the best of his or her ability and document that sublethal amounts of medication are accessible to the patient and that the supply of medication has been used up before more is prescribed. The clinician must monitor the medication adequately for the duration of the therapy and should either discontinue the medication or attempt to do so at appropriate intervals, or document in the clinical record the reasons for the decision not to do this.

Examples of behavior that may increase medicolegal risk include failing to prescribe medication for a condition for which most practitioners would prescribe medication, prescribing an inappropriate drug for the diagnosis, using an unsatisfactory rationale to justify the choice of drug, administering an inappropriate dosage for the disorder (e.g., subtherapeutic levels of a tricyclic), administering medication by an inappropriate route (e.g., continuing to give medication intramuscularly when it is no longer indicated or necessary) or polypharmacy, the simultaneous use of two or more similar drugs, usually from the same class (as opposed to copharmacy, which is the simultaneous use of drugs from different classes, such as an antiparkinsonian drug and an antipsychotic). A patient's use of prescribed medication to attempt or successfully complete a suicide may also result in legal action.

Deviating from a Manufacturer's Labeling of a Drug

This book discusses many uses of psychoactive medications that are different from those formally recommended by the manufacturer or approved of by the FDA for advertising as safe and effective. Many of these unlabeled uses are medically accepted, but others are not yet common medical practice. Deviating from usual clinical practice increases the risk of legal action. Although legally permissible, using FDA-approved drugs for non-FDA-approved indications and using FDA-approved drugs for approved indications in children below the age limit for which they are approved may increase the potential for liability. Similarly, not adhering to the recommendations of the drug manufacturer (in the package insert or as reprinted in the PDR)—for example, exceeding recommended dosages—should alert the clinician to carefully document the rationale for doing so. In general, however, clinicians are on solid ground if they have assessed the risk/benefit ratio for prescribing a medication for a non-FDA-approved indication and have documented a scientifically reasonable rationale for choosing a particular drug over other possible treatments in the medical record.

In clinical practice, standard treatments and unlabeled (non-FDA-approved) but clinically accepted treatments that may be efficacious with less risk almost always should be tried before less clinically accepted or riskier medications are used. Concurrence of a consultant and appropriate psychopharmacological references supporting such use may be helpful when the unlabeled use is not commonly accepted (Nurcombe, 1990). As a general principle, the more novel the treatment or uncertain the risk/benefit ratio, the more severely disabling should be the condition for which it is used.

Issues Concerned with Documenting Ongoing Appropriate Attention to Medication and Related Matters in the Clinical Record

The patient's clinical record should reflect continued appropriate monitoring of the medication's efficacy, presence or absence of untoward effects, results of laboratory tests or other procedures (e.g., ECG) used to monitor untoward effects, justifications for increases or decreases in dosage or changes in times of administration, decisions to employ a drug holiday or discontinue medication, and the consequences of discontinuing medication, including any change in symptomatology, reexacerbation of symptoms, rebound effects, or withdrawal syndromes such as a withdrawal dyskinesia.

When patients are hospitalized, it is important for the clinician to address in the progress notes not only his or her own observations of the patient but also those of other disciplines who have reported or recorded behaviors or symptoms that may indicate untoward effects of medication (e.g., unsteadiness of gait reported by a nurse or falling asleep in class reported by a teacher).

Most authorities recommend that children and adolescents who are receiving psychoactive medication should have it discontinued or at least tapered down periodically, typically within 6 months to at most a year, to ascertain whether or not it is still needed or whether a lower dose might be sufficient. That this has been done should be documented in the chart, and if the clinician delays this unusually, the reason should be clearly explained in the chart (e.g., the previous attempt resulted in a severe relapse of symptoms that were difficult to control in a schizophrenic adolescent, or a clinical decision has been reached to delay an attempt to lower or discontinue medication until the completion of the school year as functioning has been marginal even though somewhat improved with medication). Decisions such as these should also be discussed with the parents and patient and their consents obtained.

Nurcombe's (1990) review of medicolegal aspects of the entire practice of child and adolescent psychiatry, including specific court cases and decisions, is recommended to the interested reader. Popper (1987a) has written an interesting chapter on ethical considerations of the relationship between obtaining consent for the use of medication from parents and children and adolescents and incomplete or unknown medical knowledge of the risks and long-term effects of psychoactive medication used during childhood and adolescence.

BASELINE ASSESSMENTS PRIOR TO INITIATION OF MEDICATION

All patients should have a complete medical history and physical and neurological examinations. This is essential to identify any organic factors contributing to the psychiatric symptomatology and any coexisting medical abnormalities. In addition, all drugs may cause untoward physical and psychological effects; hence a baseline examination prior to initiation of psychopharmacotherapy should be mandatory.

Because relatively little information is available concerning the long-term untoward effects of psychoactive drugs on the growth and development of children and adolescents, as well as the potential medicolegal ramifications, particularly when drugs are used for non-FDA-approved indications, it is recommended that the premedication work-up should be reasonably comprehensive. The reader who wishes a more detailed review of laboratory tests and diagnostic procedures applicable to general psychiatry than is provided below is referred to the helpful book by Rosse et al. (1989).

Physical Examination

This should include recording baseline temperature, pulse rate, respiration rate, and blood pressure. Height and weight should be entered on standardized growth charts, such as the National Center for Health Statistics Growth Charts (Hamill et al., 1976), so that serial measurements and percentiles may be plotted over time. A pregnancy test should be considered for any adolescent who might be pregnant, as drugs may have known or unknown adverse effects on the developing fetus. As a related issue, if an adolescent is considered to be at significant risk for becoming pregnant despite birth control counseling, certain medications (e.g., lithium) should not be prescribed if at all possible.

Laboratory Tests and Diagnostic Procedures

The following are frequently recommended premedication laboratory tests and diagnostic procedures. Some of these tests may already have been done as a part of the pediatric/medical evaluation that should be a part of any comprehensive psychiatric evaluation. These tests will be addressed more specifically under each class of medications or, if appropriate, for specific drugs when they are discussed. Obviously, the premedication work-up will be influenced by and should be modified to accommodate any particular abnormal findings in the medical history or examination, such as renal, thyroid, and cardiac abnormalities, or by any initial abnormal laboratory results themselves.

Laboratory tests routinely or frequently recommended as part of a comprehensive complete pediatric examination and/or premedication work-up include the following:

1. complete blood count (CBC), differential, and hematocrit
2. urinalysis

3. blood urea nitrogen (BUN) level
4. serum electrolyte levels for sodium (Na^+), potassium (K^+), chloride (Cl^-), calcium (Ca^{++}), and phosphate (PO_4), and carbon dioxide (CO_2) content
5. liver function tests: aspartate aminotransferase (AST) or serum glutamic oxaloacetic transaminase (SGOT), alanine aminotransferase (ALT) or serum glutamic pyruvic transaminase (SGPT), alkaline phosphatase, lactic dehydrogenase (LDH), and bilirubin (total and indirect)
6. serum lead level determination in children under 7 years of age and in older children when indicated

Other laboratory tests are often recommended prior to using specific psychoactive medications:

Thyroid Function Tests

Thyroid function tests (thyroxine [T_4], triiodothyronine resin uptake [T_3RU], and thyroid-stimulating hormone [TSH] or thyrotropin) are recommended prior to the use of tricyclic antidepressants and lithium. Abnormal thyroid function can aggravate cardiac arrhythmias that may occur as an untoward effect of tricyclic antidepressants (PDR, 1990). Lithium has been reported to cause hypothyroidism, with lower T_3 and T_4 levels and elevated I^{131} uptake.

Kidney Function Tests

Because of reported untoward effects of lithium carbonate on the kidney, baseline evaluation of kidney function should be determined. Jefferson et al. (1987) suggest that a baseline serum creatinine and urinalysis are usually adequate and that more extensive testing (e.g., creatinine clearance, 24-hour urine volume, and maximal urine osmolality) is not practical or necessary for most patients.

Special Tests

Electrocardiogram

A baseline ECG should be recorded prior to the administration of tricyclic antidepressants (with the usual exception of low doses for treatment of enuresis), as clinically important cardiac abnormalities may occur, especially at higher serum levels. The ECG should be monitored with dose increases and periodically thereafter if tricyclics are used and doses over 2.5 mg/kg are given (see below under "Tricyclic Antidepressants").

Lithium may also cause cardiac abnormalities, and an ECG is recommended prior to initiating therapy. Although it may be considered optional in young, healthy subjects, it should be mandatory in any person with a history of or clinical findings suggestive of cardiovascular disease.

Electroencephalogram

An EEG may be considered if antipsychotics, tricyclic antidepressants, or lithium will be administered, as all these drugs have been associated with either lowered threshold to seizures or other EEG changes. This would include patients who have a history of seizure disorder, who are on an antiepileptic for a seizure disorder, or who may be at risk for seizures (e.g., following brain surgery or head injury).

Baseline Behavioral Assessment

Clinical Observations

Baseline observations and careful characterizations of both behavior and target symptoms must be recorded in the clinical record. These should include direct observations by the clinician in the waiting room, office, playroom, and/or on the ward, as well as those reported by other reliable observers to occur in other locations, such as the home and school. It is important to include usual eating and sleeping patterns, as these may be altered by many drugs. These observations should be described both qualitatively and quantitatively (amplitude and frequency) and the circumstances in which they occur noted in the clinical record.

It is also essential to record an accurate baseline rating in the clinical record before beginning psychopharmacotherapy in children or adolescents who have existing abnormal movements or who are at risk for developing them (e.g., patients diagnosed with autistic disorder or severe mental retardation and/or patients who will be treated with antipsychotics). This is necessary both to follow the patient's clinical course and to be able to differentiate among recrudescence of preexisting involuntary movements, stereotypies, and mannerisms and any subsequent withdrawal dyskinesias or new stereotypies that may occur when medication, particularly an antipsychotic, is discontinued. The availability of these longitudinal data becomes even more critical if the treating physician changes.

Although the baseline data can be documented in the clinician's records, the use of a rating scale such as the Abnormal

Involuntary Movement Scale (AIMS) ("Rating Scales," 1985) that assesses abnormal movements is strongly recommended.

To be able to assess the efficacy of a specific medication, a baseline observation period, with reasonably stable or worsening target symptoms, is necessary. Other than in emergency situations (e.g., a violent, physically assaultive, and/or severely psychotic teenager), observation of the patient for a minimum of 7 to 10 days is recommended before initiating pharmacotherapy. For inpatients, this will permit assessment of the combined effects of hospitalization and a therapeutic milieu and the removal of the identified patient from his or her living situation upon the patient's psychopathology and symptoms. For outpatients, this observation period will give the clinician an opportunity to see the effect of the clinical contact and assessment on the symptom expression of the patient and the psychodynamic equilibrium of the family. During this observation period, many children and adolescents, both inpatients and outpatients, will improve sufficiently so that psychopharmacotherapy will no longer be indicated.

Rating Scales

Rating scales are an essential component of psychopharmacological research. They provide a means of recording serial qualitative and quantitative measurements of behaviors and their interrater reliability can be determined. Two of the most influential publications concerning rating scales and psychopharmacological research in children are the *Psychopharmacology Bulletin*'s special issue *Pharmacotherapy of Children* (1973) and its 1985 issue featuring "Rating Scales and Assessment Instruments for Use in Pediatric Psychopharmacology Research" ("Rating Scales, 1985).

Although rating scales are also valuable in nonresearch settings, they tend to be used less in clinical practice. Perhaps those most frequently used are the various Conners rating instruments: Conners Teacher Questionnaire (CTQ), Conners Parent-Teacher Questionnaire, Conners Parent Questionnaire (CPQ) (*Psychopharmacology Bulletin*, 1973). The abbreviated Conners Parent-Teacher Questionnaire (CAPTQ), reproduced as Figure 2.1, is useful in helping to identify patients who have ADHD and to record serial ratings that provide good periodic estimates of the clinical efficacy of medication in the classroom and home environments. The CAPTQ can be completed in a short time as it has

DEPARTMENT OF HEALTH, EDUCATION, AND WELFARE
HEALTH SERVICES AND MENTAL HEALTH ADMINISTRATION
NATIONAL INSTITUTE OF MENTAL HEALTH

CONNERS PARENT-TEACHER QUESTIONNAIRE

INSTRUCTIONS: Listed below are items concerning children's behavior or the problems they sometimes have. Read each item carefully and decide how much you think this child has been bothered by this problem *at this time:* NOT AT ALL, JUST A LITTLE, PRETTY MUCH, or VERY MUCH. Indicate your choice by circling the number in the appropriate column to the right of each item.

ANSWER ALL ITEMS

	Not at All	Just a Little	Pretty Much	Very Much
1. Restless (overactive)	0	1	2	3
2. Excitable, impulsive	0	1	2	3
3. Disturbs other children	0	1	2	3

	None 0	Minor 1	Moderate 2	Severe 3
4. Fails to finish things he starts (short attention span)	0	1	2	3
5. Fidgeting	0	1	2	3
6. Inattentive, distractable	0	1	2	3
7. Demands must be met immediately; frustrated	0	1	2	3
8. Cries	0	1	2	3
9. Mood changes quickly	0	1	2	3
10. Temper outbursts (explosive and unpredictable behavior)	0	1	2	3

How serious a problem do you think this child has at this time?

Figure 2.1. Conners Parent-Teacher Questionnaire. (Modified, from Department of Health, Education, and Welfare, Health Services and Mental Health Administration, National Institutes of Health.)

only 11 items. The first 10 items are common to the CTQ and the CPQ; the eleventh item is an overall estimate of the degree of seriousness of the child's problem at the time of the rating and is not included in the following discussion of scoring. A total score of 15 on the first 10 items has been used widely in research as the cut-off for 2 standard deviations above the mean, and subjects scoring 15 or more points have been considered hyperactive (Sleator, 1986). The mean value of the 10 items of the CAPTQ yields a score comparable to Factor IV, the hyperactivity index, of the CTQ, and a 0.5-point or more decrease in the mean (or of 5 points in the total score on the first 10 items of the CAPTQ) generally indicates that medication is effecting a meaningful improvement (Greenhill, 1990.)

The AIMS (Fig. 2.2) is a 12-item scale designed to record in detail the occurrence of dyskinetic movements. Abnormal involuntary movements are rated on a 5-point scale from 0 to 4, with 0 being none, 1 being minimal or extreme normal, 2 being mild, 3 being moderate, and 4 being severe. If a procedure is used to activate the movements (e.g., having the patient tap his or her thumb with each finger as rapidly as possible for 10 to 15 seconds separately with the right and then the left hand), movements are rated 1 point lower than those occurring spontaneously. Seven of the items rate abnormal involuntary movements in specific topographies: 4 items concern facial and oral movements, 2 items concern extremity movements, and 1 item concerns trunk movements. Three items are global ratings: 2 by the clinician concern the overall severity of the abnormal movements and the estimated degree of incapacity from them, and a third records the patient's own degree of awareness of the abnormal movements. Using the AIMS will also make it less likely that an area that should be assessed will be omitted inadvertently and will also provide quantitative ratings for following the clinical course. Having a baseline and subsequent AIMS ratings available is most helpful to the initial treating physician in assessing any changes in baseline abnormal involuntary movements increases, decrements, or changes in topography during the course of active treatment with psychoactive medication, as well as during periods of withdrawal from medication. These ratings are often essential to differentiate preexisting abnormal involuntary movements from withdrawal dyskinesias. Such ratings are even more helpful when other physicians may assume the treatment of the patient at a future time.

Medicating the Patient

Selecting the Initial Medication

In general, it is recommended that an FDA-approved standard medication for the patient's age, diagnosis, and target symptoms be chosen initially whenever it is likely to be clinically efficacious. Factors such as selecting the drug with the least risk of serious untoward effects; known previous response(s) of the patient to psychotropic medication; the responses of siblings, parents, and other relatives with psychiatric illnesses to psychotropic medication; family history (e.g., a history of Tourette's disorder); and the clinician's own previous experience in using the medication should also be weighed in choosing the initial and, if necessary, subsequent drugs.

Generic versus Trade Preparations

There has been controversy in the literature on the merits of brand names, usually the initial, patented preparations of a medication, and generic preparations, which typically enter the market after exclusive patent rights expire and cost considerably less than the brand-name product. Although the active ingredients in the various preparations should be pharmaceutically equivalent, the inert ingredients and the manufacturing processes may vary and hence the bioavailability of a drug may be significantly different among various preparations.

Many states now permit substitution of generic drugs for drugs prescribed by brand name under specified conditions. New York State, for example, requires all prescription forms to have imprinted on them "This prescription will be filled generically unless prescriber writes 'daw' [dispense as written] in the box below." New York State publishes a book, *Safe, Effective and Therapeutically Equivalent Prescription Drugs*, listing approved preparations of various prescription drugs. Pharmacists are directed to "substitute a less expensive drug product containing the same active ingredients, dosage form and strength" as the drug originally prescribed, if available (New York State Department of Health, 1988, p. iii). The book recognizes differences in bioavailability among products. For example, for chlorpromazine it does not authorize substitution of oral solid immediate-release products because of potential bioequivalence problems.

The FDA Center for Drug Evaluation and Research publishes

DEPARTMENT OF HEALTH, EDUCATION, AND WELFARE
PUBLIC HEALTH SERVICE
ALCOHOL, DRUG ABUSE, AND MENTAL HEALTH ADMINISTRATION
NATIONAL INSTITUTE OF MENTAL HEALTH

ABNORMAL INVOLUNTARY MOVEMENT SCALE (AIMS)

INSTRUCTIONS: Complete Examination Procedure (see pp. 36–37) before making ratings.

MOVEMENT RATINGS: Rate highest severity observed. Rate movements that occur upon activation one *less than* those observed spontaneously.

Code:
0 = None
1 = Minimal, may be extreme normal
2 = Mild
3 = Moderate
4 = Severe

FACIAL AND ORAL MOVEMENTS:		(Circle One)				
1.	**Muscles of Facial Expression** e.g., movements of forehead, eyebrows, periorbital area, cheeks; include frowning, blinking, smiling, grimacing	0	1	2	3	4
2.	**Lips and Perioral Area** e.g., puckering, pouting, smacking	0	1	2	3	4
3.	**Jaw** e.g., biting, clenching, chewing, mouth opening, lateral movement	0	1	2	3	4
4.	**Tongue** Rate only increase in movement both in and out of mouth, NOT inability to sustain movement	0	1	2	3	4

EXTREMITY MOVEMENTS:	5.	**Upper** *(arms, wrists, hands, fingers)* Include choreic movements, (i.e., rapid, objectively purposeless, irregular, spontaneous), athetoid movements (i.e., slow, irregular, complex, serpentine). Do NOT include tremor (i.e., repetitive, regular, rhythmic)		0	1	2	3	4
	6.	**Lower** *(legs, knees, ankles, toes)* e.g., lateral knee movement, foot tapping, heel dropping, foot squirming, inversion and eversion of foot		0	1	2	3	4
TRUNK MOVEMENTS:	7.	**Neck, shoulders, hips** e.g., rocking, twisting, squirming, pelvic gyrations		0	1	2	3	4
GLOBAL JUDGE-MENTS:	8.	**Severity of abnormal movements**	None, normal / Minimal / Mild / Moderate / Severe	0	1	2	3	4
	9.	**Incapacitation due to abnormal movements**	None, normal / Minimal / Mild / Moderate / Severe	0	1	2	3	4
	10.	**Patient's awareness of abnormal movements** Rate only patient's report	No awareness / Aware, no distress / Aware, mild distress / Aware, moderate distress / Aware, severe distress	0	1	2	3	4
DENTAL STATUS:	11.	**Current problems with teeth and/or dentures**	No / Yes	0	1			
	12.	**Does patient usually wear dentures?**	No / Yes	0	1			

(Continued)

Figure 2.2. Abnormal Involuntary Movement Scale (AIMS). (Modified, from Department of Health, Education, and Welfare, Public Health Service, Alcohol, Drug Abuse, and Mental Health Administration, National Institute of Mental Health.)

EXAMINATION PROCEDURE

Either before or after completing the Examination Procedure observe the patient unobtrusively, at rest (e.g., in waiting room).

The chair to be used in this examination should be a hard, firm one without arms.

1. Ask patient whether there is anything in his/her mouth (i.e., gum, candy, etc.) and if there is, to remove it.

2. Ask patient about the <u>current</u> condition of his/her teeth. Ask patient if he/she wears dentures. Do teeth or dentures bother patient <u>now</u>?

3. Ask patient whether he/she notices any movements in mouth, face, hands, or feet. If yes, ask to describe and to what extent they <u>currently</u> bother patient or interfere with his/her activities.

4. Have patient sit in chair with hands on knees, legs slightly apart, and feet flat on floor. (Look at entire body for movements while in this position).

5. Ask patient to sit with hands hanging unsupported. If male, between legs, if female and wearing a dress, hanging over knees. (Observe hands and other body areas.)

6. Ask patient to open mouth. (Observe tongue at rest within mouth.) Do this twice.

7. Ask patient to protrude tongue. (Observe abnormalities of tongue movement.) Do this twice.

8. Ask patient to tap thumb, with each finger, as rapidly as possible for 10–15 seconds; separately with right hand, then with left hand. (Observe facial and leg movements.)

9. Flex and extend patient's left and right arms (one at a time). (Note any rigidity and rate on DOTES.)

10. Ask patient to stand up. (Observe in profile. Observe all body areas again, hips included.)

■ 11. Ask patient to extend both arms outstretched in front with palms down. (Observe trunk, legs, and mouth.)

■ 12. Have patient walk a few paces, turn, and walk back to chair. (Observe hands and gait.) Do this twice.

■ Activated movements

Figure 2.2. Abnormal Involuntary Movement Scale (continued).

a book, *Approved Drug Products with Therapeutic Equivalence Evaluations* (the "Orange Book"), which is a list of drugs, both prescription and nonprescription, approved by the FDA on the basis of safety and effectiveness. The list gives the FDA's evaluations of the therapeutic equivalence of prescription drugs that are available from multiple sources. It classifies drug preparations into two basic categories: A ratings, which are given to drug products that the FDA considers to be therapeutically equivalent to other pharmaceutically equivalent products, where there are no known or suspected bioequivalence problems or where actual or potential problems are thought to have been satisfactorily resolved; and B ratings, which are drug products that the FDA does not at this time consider to be therapeutically equivalent to other pharmaceutically equivalent products.

The 1988 FDA "Orange Book," for example, rates preparations of chlorpromazine for oral administration as "BP," indicating that there are potential bioequivalence problems among these preparations. Oral preparations of nortriptyline are rated "BD," indicating that there have been documented bioequivalence problems when a pharmaceutically equivalent drug from another source was substituted. Dubovsky (1987) reported a case of severe nortriptyline intoxication due to changing from a generic to a trade preparation, which seemed to result from the significantly greater bioavailability of the trade preparation.

These comments are not a recommendation for any preparation over any other but are meant to alert the clinician that different preparations of the same medication of the same strength may have different bioavailabilities, and that when they are substituted for one another, there is a potential for significant clinical repercussions. If prescriptions are written that may be filled with various generic preparations, it is prudent for the physician to inform the patient or responsible adult that if the medication is different when refilled to inform him or her and to note any changes in symptoms or feelings after switching to a new preparation. Although changes in manufacturer may occur at times even when prescriptions are filled at the same pharmacy, the likelihood of a change in manufacturer increases when different pharmacies are used. If a patient runs out of medication while traveling and has to obtain medication from a new source, a change of manufacturer may be more likely. Hence it is worthwhile to remember to ascertain that a patient has sufficient medication before going off to summer camp or traveling.

Standard and Nonstandard Treatments

In this book, standard treatments will be considered those treatments that have been approved by the FDA for advertising and interstate commerce. This implies that the drug has demonstrated clinical efficacy and that its use is substantially safe. The FDA's legal authority over how marketed drugs are used, the dosages employed, and related matters is limited to regulating what the manufacturer may recommend and must disclose in the package insert or labeling. "The prescription of a drug for an unlabeled indication is entirely proper if based on rational scientific theory, reliable medical opinion, or controlled clinical trials" (American Medical Association, 1986, p. 9).

Over the past 2 decades, a substantial body of clinical and investigational data has accumulated on using FDA-approved drugs to treat children below the recommended age for use (e.g., imipramine to treat major depressive disorder in children under 12 years of age), using FDA-approved drugs to treat children and adolescents for non-FDA-approved (nonlabeled) indications (e.g., lithium to treat aggressive conduct disorder in any age group and tricyclic antidepressants to treat ADHD), and using drugs not approved by the FDA for any indication (investigational drugs) to treat psychiatric disorders in children and adolescents. For example, until it was recently approved by the FDA for treating obsessive-compulsive disorder in patients at least 10 years of age, clomipramine was an investigational drug.

Lithium and the tricyclic antidepressants are, at present, the most clinically important of the FDA-approved drugs used for nonapproved indications in children and adolescents. For example, there appears to be a growing consensus among child psychiatrists that the risks of using lithium and some of the tricyclic antidepressants for non-FDA-approved indications are often preferable to using antipsychotics that increase the risks of impairing cognitive functioning and carry significant risk of producing tardive dyskinesia. This will be discussed in more detail in the specific drug section of the book.

Drug Interactions

Many psychoactive drugs have significant interactions with other medications. It is essential to ascertain any medication, prescription or otherwise, that the patient may be taking concurrently and to evaluate the potential interaction.

As part of the medical history, inquiries should be made about all medications, including those prescribed by other physicians, over-the-counter preparations used even occasionally by the patient, and, as appropriate, alcohol and illicit or recreational drug use. Parents or caretakers and patients as appropriate to their age and mental abilities should be instructed to inform any physicians who may treat them while they are on psychoactive medication of the medications that are currently being taken. Similarly, patients the clinician is treating with psychoactive medication should be instructed to report back at the next appointment if a physician prescribes them any other medication or if they take any other drugs, over the counter or illicit, on their own initiative.

If substance abuse is known or suspected, screening of urine and/or blood for toxic substances may be indicated.

Drug interactions are discussed for each of the classes of psychoactive drugs. An attempt has been made to emphasize the most important interactions and those interactions most likely to be encountered by the physician who is treating psychiatrically disturbed children and adolescents.

It is beyond the scope of this book to review all possible drug interactions. It is the prescribing physician's responsibility to attempt to determine any other drugs his or her patient is taking and to assess any potentially adverse interactions of the medications before prescribing a new medication. The package insert, current PDR (1990), current *Drug Interactions and Side Effects Index* (1990), *Drug Interactions in Psychiatry* (Ciraulo et al., 1989), or other suitable reference should be consulted. When appropriate and with the patient's consent, any other physicians treating the patient should be contacted so that a comprehensive treatment regimen that addresses safely both the psychiatric and the medical disorders of the patient may be mutually developed.

Regulating the Medication

Selecting the Initial Dosage

It is recommended that the treating physician initially prescribe a low dose, which will be either ineffective or inadequate for most patients. Although this cautious approach may lengthen the time necessary to reach a therapeutic dose, it is worthwhile for several reasons. First, pharmacokinetics vary not only among various age groups but also among individuals of a specific age. For genetic and other reasons, some individuals may be highly sensitive and responsive to a given medication or slow metabolizers, while others may be relatively resistant or nonresponsive. By beginning with a low dose, one will avoid starting at a dose that is already in excess of the optimal therapeutic dose for a few patients, and those children and adolescents who are good responders at low dosages of medication will not be missed. If the initial dose is too high, the therapeutic range for these low-dose responders will not be explored and only untoward effects, which may at times even be confused with worsening of target symptoms, will be seen. Hence a potentially beneficial medication may be needlessly excluded. For example, with stimulants a worsening of behavior may occur when optimal therapeutic doses for a specific patient have been exceeded. Second, with some drugs (e.g., methylphenidate) there is no significant relationship between serum level and clinical response. Third, excessive initial dosage may also cause behavioral toxicity, particularly in younger children. Behavioral toxicity may occur before other side effects and includes such symptoms as worsening of target symptoms, hyperactivity or hypoactivity, aggressiveness, increased irritability, mood changes, apathy and decreased verbal productions (Campbell et al., 1985). Fourth, some untoward effects of the drug may be eliminated or minimized; for example, acute dystonic reactions of antipsychotics and some untoward effects of lithium carbonate appear to be related in many cases to both serum levels and the rapidity of increase in serum level, and sedation may be less of a problem if dosage is increased gradually (Green et al., 1985).

Timing of Drug Administration

Scheduling Dosages

Times chosen for administration of the drug and the number of times the drug is administered per day should be related to the pharmacokinetics of the drug; for example, stimulants are most frequently given around breakfast and lunch, while antipsychotics may initially be given three or four times daily to reduce the risk of sedation and acute dystonic reactions. Once dosage has been stabilized, it may be clinically more convenient and may sometimes increase compliance if medications that have longer half-lives are administered only once or twice daily.

Pharmacokinetics and developmentally determined pharmacodynamic factors must still take precedence over convenience. For example, it may be possible to give the entire daily dose of an antipsychotic at bedtime to children and adolescents, whereas because younger children metabolize tricyclic antidepressants differently from the way adolescents and adults metabolize them and may be more sensitive to cardiotoxic effects, it is recommended that these drugs continue to be administered to children and younger adolescents in divided doses.

Drug Holidays

Because of the untoward effects of medication and their known and unknown effects on the growth, maturation, and development of children and adolescents, it is universally agreed that it is prudent to use medication in as low doses and for as short a time as is clinically expedient. For some children, "drug holidays" may be a useful means of minimizing the cumulative amount of medication taken over time. The feasibility and type of drug holidays vary with diagnosis and the severity of the disorder.

When stimulant medication is needed primarily to improve behavior (increase attention span and decrease hyperactivity and sometimes conduct problems) for classroom functioning as with some ADHD children, it is often possible to withhold medication holidays and weekends and during school vacations, including the entire summer. This is particularly important if there appears to be evidence of any suppression of height and weight percentiles, as there may be catch-up or compensatory growth following discontinuation of stimulant medication.

Sometimes parents find that their hyperactive child is not a serious management problem without medication at home but that difficulties arise when the child accompanies them on a shopping excursion or goes to a birthday party. In cases like this, where the parents' judgment can be trusted and medication is not used as a punishment, an understanding with the parents and child that medication may be used occasionally on weekends or vacations in situations that are particularly difficult for the child may be therapeutically indicated.

There is reasonable concern about the possibility of an irreversible tardive dyskinesia's developing in children and adolescents who receive long-term therapy with antipsychotic medication. There is some evidence that the development of tardive dyskinesia may be associated with both the total amount of antipsychotic ingested and the duration of treatment, although constitutional vulnerabilities to developing tardive dyskinesia also appear to play an important role (Jeste & Wyatt, 1982). Consequently, possible means of reducing the total amount of antipsychotic consumed may be clinically important in reducing the likelihood of developing tardive dyskinesia.

Newton et al. (1989) compared 6-week periods of haloperidol daily versus with 6-week periods of haloperidol with repeated weekly 2-day drug holidays in a cross-over experiment with seven older adult schizophrenic patients. Serum haloperidol levels were reduced by about 25% during holiday periods, with no significant change in mental status, severity of psychiatric symptoms, or scores on scales rating movement disorders.

Similarly, Perry et al. (1989) reported on 52 child outpatients aged 2.3 years to 7.9 years diagnosed with infantile autism, full syndrome, who were treated with haloperidol for 6 months. The subjects were assigned on a random basis in a double-blind protocol to receive haloperidol continuously (daily) or discontinuously (5 days per week with 2 contiguous days of placebo). There was no significant clinical difference between the groups, and in both groups children who had symptoms of irritability, angry and labile affect, and uncooperativeness responded best. The incidence of untoward effects, including tardive and withdrawal dyskinesia, did not vary significantly between the two groups.

If additional studies continue to find no significant difference in therapeutic efficacy between antipsychotics administered 7 days versus 5 days per week, this may become the preferred method of long-term maintenance to decrease the total cumulative amount of antipsychotic ingested over time, in the hope of diminishing the incidence of irreversible tardive dyskinesia; it also has the additional benefit of reducing the cost of medication by nearly 30%.

Dosage Increases

Changes in medication level should be based on the clinical response of the patient, and the rationale for each change should be documented in the clinical record. Knowledge of the characteristic time frame of response for a particular drug and diagnosis should influence these decisions. Thus the clinician may increase dosage once or twice weekly in some cases, when using stimulants or neuroleptics. On the other hand, the clinical efficacy of tricyclic antidepressants may not be fully apparent for several weeks when used to treat major depressive disorder. Once daily dosage has reached a level that is usually associated with clinical response, increasing the dose because of a failure to respond during the first 2 or 3 weeks of treatment is not psychophar-macologically sound practice unless serum drug levels are being monitored and are felt to be in the subtherapeutic range.

Titration of Medication

The goal of the clinician is to achieve meaningful therapeutic benefits for the patient with the fewest possible untoward effects. Here again it is recommended that risks versus benefits be as-sessed. To do so scientifically, however, it is necessary to explore the dose range of a patient's response. Hence unless there are extenuating circumstances, it is usually advisable to continue raising the dose level until one of the following events occurs:

1. Entirely adequate symptom control is established.
2. The upper limit of the recommended dosage (or higher level if commonly accepted) has been reached.
3. Untoward effects that preclude a further increase in dose have occurred.
4. After a measurable improvement in target symptoms, a plateau in improvement or a worsening of symptoms occurs with fur-ther increases in dose.

Unless this is done, an injustice may be done to the patient. This occurs most frequently when there is some behavioral im-provement and the treating clinician stabilizes the dosage at that point. Further significant improvement that might have occurred had a higher dose been given is missed. It is recommended that the next higher dose or two should be explored. If there is signifi-cant additional improvement, the therapist in consultation with the patient and his or her parents can make a judgment as to whether the benefits from this outweigh the risks from the addi-tional dosage.

Determining the Optimal Dose

Once the upper limit of the therapeutic dose range has been explored for a specific patient, the lowest possible dose that pro-duces the desired effects should be determined. This is consid-ered the optimal dose for a specific patient. In clinical practice, this may be a compromise, and amelioration of target symptoms to an acceptable degree may occur only when some untoward effects are also present.

In those cases where either no significant therapeutic benefit occurs or untoward effects prevent employment of a clinically meaningful therapeutic dose, a trial of a different medication must be considered.

Untoward Effects (Side Effects)

All drugs, including placebos, have untoward effects or side effects. Actually, if one excludes allergic and idiosyncratic reactions, many untoward effects are as much a characteristic of the pharmacological make-up of a specific drug and are as predictable as the drug's therapeutic effects. Individual patients may vary as much in their development of side effects to a drug as in their therapeutic responses to it.

It is sometimes useful to think of untoward effects as the "unwanted effects" of the drug for the specific patient and therapeutic indication. For a different patient and situation an untoward or side effect will actually become the desired therapeutic action of the drug. For example, sedation, which may be an untoward effect when a benzodiazepine is prescribed for anxiolysis, is the desired result when a benzodiazepine is prescribed as a soporific. Similarly, appetite suppression is usually an undesired effect of stimulants prescribed for ADHD but the action of choice when they are used in treating exogenous obesity.

Many untoward effects are related to dose or serum levels, but others are not. They may occur almost immediately (e.g., an acute dystonic reaction) or be delayed for years (e.g., tardive dyskinesia). They may be life threatening or fatal, or relatively innocuous. There is also evidence that the untoward effects of a specific drug may differ according to age and/or diagnosis of the subjects. For example, haloperidol produced excessive sedation in hospitalized school-age aggressive conduct-disordered children on doses of 0.04 to 0.21 mg/kg/day (Campbell et al., 1984b) but not in preschoolers with autistic disorder on doses of 0.019 to 0.217 mg/kg/day (Anderson et al., 1984).

A thorough knowledge of the most important and frequent side effects of the medications considered is essential and will often play a decisive role in which medication is selected and/or which dosage is scheduled. For example, if a schizophrenic youngster has insomnia, the clinician may select a low-potency antipsychotic and adjust the dosage schedule so that any sedation will aid the child in falling asleep. As an added benefit, risk of an acute dystonic reaction is lower than if a high-potency antipsychotic had been chosen.

Likewise, the management of unwanted effects is a vital component of pharmacotherapy. In clinical practice, careful attention to unwanted effects and flexibility as to the time and amounts of specific doses may enable one to obtain a satisfactory clinical result with a minimal or acceptable level of untoward effects that is not possible if a fixed dosage schedule is used, as in some research protocols. Thus one can adjust medication levels slowly and in small increments, or one can divide doses unequally over the day (e.g., giving more in the morning or more before bed, or the entire daily dose at bedtime).

The clinician must remember that the ability to understand untoward effects and verbalize unusual sensations, feelings, or discomfort not only varies among individual children but is developmentally determined. Younger children spontaneously report untoward effects less frequently than older children. Hence the younger the child, the more essential it becomes for caretakers to be actively looking for untoward effects and for the physician to ask the patient about untoward effects in language appropriate to the understanding of the child.

It is essential that the clinician examine the patient for the development of side effects frequently during the period when the medication is being regulated, at regular intervals during maintenance therapy, and during scheduled periodic withdrawals of the medication. For example, with antipsychotics one should look particularly for sedation and extrapyramidal side effects, the development of abnormal movements, and, during drug withdrawal periods, any evidence of a withdrawal dyskinesia. Completion of the AIMS as described above is recommended as an aid in quantifying and following abnormal movements over time.

Monitoring of Serum Levels of Drugs and/or Their Metabolites

Morselli et al. (1983) and Gualtieri et al. (1984a) have reviewed the pharmacokinetics of psychoactive drugs used in child and adolescent psychiatry and the clinical relevance of determining their serum or blood levels. Determining blood or plasma levels of drugs and/or their metabolites is most useful when accurate measurements of all significant active metabolites of a drug are available and there is a known relationship between the clinical effects of the drug and serum concentration (Gualtieri et al., 1984a).

Clinically, the monitoring of serum levels is useful to verify compliance and to be certain that adequate therapeutic serum levels are available (i.e., that values fall within the therapeutic window) and thus to avoid discontinuing a trial of medication before clinically effective serum levels have been reached or, conversely, to avoid inadvertently reaching toxic serum levels.

School-age children often have more efficient physiological systems for drug metabolism and excretion than adults do. As a result, doses comparable to those administered to adults, either on a total daily dose or a dose-per-unit-weight basis, may result in subtherapeutic serum levels in children and younger adolescents. This could be one factor contributing to the clinical observation that children with schizophrenia as a group appear to show less dramatic clinical improvement than adolescents and adults, when administered neuroleptics (Green, 1989). It will be necessary to measure antipsychotic serum levels to determine if this is due to subtherapeutic levels in some cases, as some children may also show clinical improvement at lower serum levels than adults (Rivera-Calimlim et al., 1979).

Meyers et al. (1980) reported the case of a 13-year-old pre-pubescent boy diagnosed as having schizophrenia who required a daily dose of haloperidol of at least 30 mg/day to reach therapeutic serum neuroleptic levels. Monitoring serum levels of antipsychotics thus may yield clinical information that is, at times, clinically extremely useful. If a child or adolescent does not have a satisfactory response to usual doses of antipsychotics, serum neuroleptic levels should be determined, if possible, before deciding to discontinue the drug.

In addition to age-related differences in pharmacokinetics, remarkable interindividual variations occur. For example, Berg et al. (1974) reported that a 14-year-old girl with bipolar manic-depressive disorder required up to 2400 mg of lithium daily to maintain serum lithium levels of 1 mEq/liter. Her father had the same disorder and also required unusually high doses of lithium to reach therapeutic levels.

At the present time, lithium is the only medication used in child and adolescent psychiatry (with the exception of antiepileptic drugs being used for control of seizures, which are not reviewed herein) for which regular determinations of serum levels are mandatory. This is reviewed below in the section on lithium carbonate. It is virtually certain that monitoring of serum levels (both drug and significant metabolites) will become increasing more important for many drugs used in child and adolescent psychiatry as their determinations become more readily available.

In current practice, for example, monitoring of drug and metabolite serum levels is of considerable practical importance in the use of the tricyclic antidepressants. This is because there is minimal correlation between dose and serum level, and serum levels are correlated significantly with clinical response and/or with potentially serious untoward effects (e.g., cardiotoxicity). For example, Puig-Antich et al. (1987) have emphasized that they found no predictors of total maintenance plasma levels, including dosage, in their prepubertal subjects treated with imipramine for major depressive disorder. They also reported that positive therapeutic response to imipramine in prepubertal children was strongly correlated with serum levels over 150 ng/ml.

Similarly, Biederman and colleagues (1989b) reported that desipramine serum levels varied an average of 16.5-fold at four different dose levels in 31 children and adolescents diagnosed with attention deficit disorder (ADD). These authors, however, found no significant linear relationship between the total daily dose or weight-corrected (mg/kg) daily dose and the steady-state serum desipramine level and any outcome measure, including clinical improvement. There was, however, a tendency for serum desipramine levels in subjects who were rated very much or much improved on the Clinical Global Improvement scale to average 60.8% higher than in unimproved subjects.

Morselli et al. (1983) also emphasized that monitoring drug plasma levels of haloperidol, chlorpromazine, imipramine, and clomipramine is particularly helpful in optimizing long-term treatment with these agents.

On the other hand, a recent detailed review of the pharmacokinetics and actions of methylphenidate concluded that "blood MPH [methylphenidate] levels are not statistically related to clinical response, nor are they likely to prove clinically helpful until this lack of correlation is understood" (Patrick et al., 1987, p. 1393).

Length of Time to Continue Medication

Children and adolescents are immature, developing organisms. Because of concerns about long-term untoward effects such as tardive and withdrawal dyskinesias and growth retardation and our inadequate knowledge of other long-term untoward effects of psychopharmacological agents on their biological and psychological maturation, there is virtually unanimous agreement that medication should be given for as short a period as possible.

The vicissitudes of the natural courses of psychiatric illnesses in children and adolescents are often not predictable for specific individuals. It is to be hoped, especially when there is a significant psychosocial etiological factor, that medication will augment the child's response to other therapeutic interventions and enhance his or her social and academic functioning, maturation, and development. Once real gains are made and internalized, the cycle of failures broken, and maladaptive patterns replaced with more appropriate ones, it may be possible to discontinue the drug and maintain therapeutic gains. Even in chronic conditions with strong biological underpinnings, such as pervasive developmental disorder, schizophrenia, and depression, the clinical course may spontaneously vary so that in some patients psychoactive medication may be reduced or even discontinued.

Periodic Withdrawal/Tapering of Medication

It is usually considered mandatory to discontinue psychotropic medications (or to attempt to do so) in child and adolescent patients on a regular basis, certainly no less frequently than every 6 months to 1 year. There may be occasional exceptions to this— for example, the long-term prophylactic use of lithium carbonate or a tricyclic antidepressant to prevent recurrences of mood disorders, or not withdrawing an antipsychotic in a child or adolescent being treated for a schizophrenia who has experienced serious relapses during prior withdrawal attempts. Whenever medication is continued beyond 6 to 12 months, it is important to document the clinical reasons for doing this in the medical record.

Withdrawal Syndromes/Untoward Effects

Rapidly metabolized drugs such as methylphenidate and amphetamines may be discontinued abruptly. However, with these drugs with short half-lives there may be some rebound effect during routine daily administration of the drug as serum levels decline in late afternoon or evening.

It is recommended that most medications, especially those with longer serum half-lives, be gradually reduced rather than stopped abruptly in order to minimize the likelihood of developing withdrawal syndromes. The clinician should continue to complete the AIMS in patients who had preexisting abnormal movements prior to initiation of medication that may have been masked or ameliorated, or who are otherwise at risk for developing abnormal movements following withdrawal. If a withdrawal dyskinesia emerges upon discontinuing an antipsychotic, every effort should be made to keep the patient off antipsychotics. Any abnormal movements should continue to be recorded on the AIMS.

Gualtieri and his colleagues reported both physical withdrawal symptoms, such as decreased appetite, nausea and vomiting, diarrhea and sweating, and acute behavioral deterioration, in about 10% of children and adolescents following their withdrawal from long-term treatment with antipsychotics. Both types of withdrawal symptoms ceased spontaneously within 8 weeks (Gualtieri et al., 1984b). It is extremely important that the clinician recognize that such symptoms may be expectable withdrawal effects and that they are not necessarily a return of premedication symptoms. The symptoms must be monitored qualitatively and quantitatively over a sufficient time to see if they diminish as one would expect with a withdrawal syndrome, or if they are an indication that the underlying psychiatric disorder still requires medication for symptom amelioration.

When tricyclics are withdrawn abruptly or too rapidly, some children experience a flu-like withdrawal syndrome resulting from cholinergic rebound. This characteristically includes gastrointestinal symptoms including nausea, abdominal discomfort and pain, vomiting, and fatigue. Tapering the medication down over a 10-day period rather than abruptly withdrawing the medication will usually avoid this or significantly diminish the withdrawal syndrome. The clinician is cautioned that in patients with poor compliance, who in essence may undergo periodic self-induced acute withdrawals, the withdrawal syndrome may be confused with untoward effects, inadequate dose levels, or worsening of the underlying psychiatric disorder.

In significant numbers of cases, after an initial treatment period of varying duration, medication may be no longer required or adequate symptom control can be maintained on a lower maintenance dose. For example, Sleator et al. (1974) administered a 1-month-long period of placebo to 28 of 42 hyperactive children who had been treated with methylphenidate for between 1 and 2 years. Eleven of the 28 were able to continue performing adequately behaviorally and academically without medication. Seventeen of the 28 showed worsening during the placebo period; of the 17, 10 functioned well when their initial dose was resumed, while 7 needed an increase in dose to maintain their original gains.

On the other hand, with the passage of time, occasionally higher doses may be required to maintain gains. This may reflect a worsening of the psychiatric disorder per se or a developmental/maturational effect, as in a child with autistic disorder who becomes both stronger and more aggressive as he or she enters adolescence. In other cases, the need for increased medication may be a consequence of an individual's normal physiological maturation's altering the drug's pharmacokinetics and/or of normal or excessive weight gain.

Section II

Specific Drug Treatments

INTRODUCTION

Child psychopharmacology is a relatively new field. The 1937 publication by Charles Bradley reporting the effects of administering racemic amphetamine sulfate (Benzedrine) to 30 children aged 5 to 14 years with various behavioral disturbances is usually considered to mark the beginning of the modern era of child psychopharmacology.

Over 20 years later, the first book concerned exclusively with issues concerning psychopharmacological research in child psychiatry, *Child Research in Psychopharmacology*, evolved out of the 1958 Conference on Child Research in Psychopharmacology sponsored by the National Institute of Mental Health (Fisher, 1959). The book contains an annotated list of 159 references of studies of the effects of psychopharmacological agents administered to children with psychiatric problems, beginning with Bradley's 1937 publication. Interestingly, M. Molitch and coworkers also published, in 1937, three papers concerning the use of amphetamine sulfate in children, including two placebo-controlled studies (Molitch & Eccles, 1937; Molitch & Poliakoff, 1937; Molitch & Sullivan, 1937). Two of the studies found that amphetamine sulfate improved scores of children on intelligence tests, and one reported that 86% of 14 enuretic boys who had not responded to placebo were dry when given increasing doses of amphetamine sulfate and reverted to bedwetting within 2 weeks after the drug was discontinued.

In the 1950s the classes of drugs currently most important in general psychiatry were introduced: the antipsychotics (chlorpromazine and other compounds), the antidepressants, and lithium carbonate. The benzodiazepines, in particular diazepam and chlordiazepoxide, were introduced into clinical psychiatric practice in the early 1960s. Because of increased difficulties in conducting psychopharmacological research and of obtaining FDA approval of the safety and efficacy of psychoactive drugs in children and younger adolescents, the investigation and introduction into clinical practice of psychoactive drugs in children has always lagged somewhat behind that for adults. Weiner and Jaffe (1985) have written a brief but interesting overview of the history of child and adolescent psychopharmacology.

The reader who wishes an in-depth review of major issues of the past decade that span the entire field of psychopharmacology is referred to *Psychopharmacology: The Third Generation of Progress* (Meltzer, 1987). Texts focusing entirely or significantly on child and adolescent psychopharmacology include those by Aman and Singh (1988), Gadow (1986a, 1986b), Campbell, Green, and Deutsch (1985), Weiner (1977, 1985), Klein, Gittelman, Quitkin, and Rifkin (1980), and Werry (1978). Green and Campbell (1987) and Campbell and Spencer (1988) have reviewed the more recent advances in child and adolescent psychopharmacology. In addition, the sections of the newly published *Treatments of Psychiatric Disorders* that discuss the psychopharmacological treatment of child and adolescent disorders merit attention (APA, 1989).

In most instances, reviews of the literature establishing the clinical efficacy and safety of standard FDA-approved treatments for the psychiatric disorders of children and adolescents are not included in this book. Readers who wish to review the research data establishing these standard treatments will find such information to be readily accessible in the texts cited above.

Part II of the present book summarizes the standard treatments but additionally focuses in greater detail on research into new and not yet approved uses of drugs in child and adolescent psychiatry and reviews these studies. Some knowledge of psychopharmacological research principles and techniques is essential to critically evaluate the data that appear in the psychiatric literature and to make informed clinical decisions on whether a trial of a particular drug is warranted for a particular patient.

Most important psychopharmacological research designs include comparison of the drug being investigated with either placebo or a drug that is an approved standard treatment for the psychiatric disorder in question. Hence it is important to have a basic understanding of placebos.

PLACEBOS

According to the *Oxford English Dictionary* (OED) (1933), the English word "placebo" was directly adopted from the Latin word meaning "I shall be pleasing or acceptable." By 1811 it was defined in *Hooper's Medical Dictionary* (OED, 1933) as "any medicine adapted more to please than benefit the patient." In 1982 the supplement to the OED added the following definition of placebo, which fairly accurately described its current use in psychopharmacological research: "A substance or procedure which a patient accepts as a medicine or therapy but which actually has no specific therapeutic activity for his condition or is prescribed in the belief that it has no such activity." Although placebos are often comprised of substances thought to be inert, in psychopharmacological research, placebos may also contain active ingredients chosen to simulate untoward effects of the drug to which the placebo is being compared. The purpose of this is to keep all participants "blind" by making it more difficult for patients and observers to distinguish between drug and placebo based solely on the drug's untoward effects.

Placebos play a crucial role in clinical psychopharmacological research by providing nonspecific treatment effects for comparison with the drug under investigation. These nonspecific psychological and physiological changes are not drug specific and may be measured by rating scales (Prien, 1988). These changes include both beneficial and untoward reactions produced by the expectations the patient or observers have about the drug, natural fluctuations in the clinical course of the disease as well as spontaneous alterations in the patient's condition that may have nothing to do with the illness under consideration, effects of the relationship between the patient and therapist as well as other medical staff, and other unknown effects.

Because of these nonspecific effects, even "inert" placebos have side effects. These commonly may include such symptoms as fatigue, tiredness, anxiety, muscle aches, nausea, diarrhea, constipation, dry mouth, dysmenorrhea, and behavioral changes such as increased or decreased aggressiveness, impulsiveness, attention span, or irritability. These are often symptoms that might appear periodically in the general population. It is the difference in incidence of these unwanted effects between placebo and drug that is important.

The most methodologically sound use of a placebo for testing a new medication is a double-blind, randomized, parallel-groups design (Prien, 1988). Stanley (1988) has written an interesting article concerning ethical and clinical considerations in the use of placebos that considered such factors as withholding medication during a placebo period and whether treatment may be ethically withheld in a placebo-controlled trial when a known treatment is available. Prien (1988) has offered six alternative study designs for use when it is not possible to use a double-blind, randomized, parallel-groups design and discussed some of their limitations. White et al. (1985) have edited a fascinating book concerning the theory, ethics, use in research and clinical practice, and mediating mechanisms of placebos.

EVALUATING RESEARCH STUDIES

Efficacy and safety are determined by a statistically significant benefit with acceptable untoward effects of the new medication as compared to placebo. Statistics, however, inform us about groups of patients, not individuals. Hence if etiologically dissimilar groups are subsumed under the same diagnosis, a few patients may truly benefit, but their improvement could be so diluted by the larger majority who did not benefit that the drug may show no statistically significant benefit. Some researchers now note if there are strong individual responders in a drug study even when there is no statistical difference between experimental and control groups. Thus individual case reports, studies of relatively small Ns, and open studies should not be summarily dismissed.

In evaluating the literature on child and adolescent psychopharmacology, it is important to remember that the fact that a drug is statistically significantly better than another drug or placebo doesn't necessarily mean that the drug is an optimal treatment for a given condition or for a specific child or adolescent. The drug may be effective only in certain environments (e.g., a laboratory) and not generalize to more ordinary circumstances, or it may improve only certain symptoms but not affect other major target symptoms to a clinically meaningful degree, or the overall improvement may be relatively modest with significant symptoms or deficits remaining. For example, Sprague and Sleator (1977) found that 0.3 mg/kg of methylphenidate produced optimal enhancement of learning short-term memory tasks in hyperkinetic children in the laboratory, but 1 mg/kg of methylphenidate produced the maximum improvement of social behavior in the classroom as shown by ratings on the Abbreviated Conners Rating Scale. Another example is that although children with autistic disorder have shown statistically significant improvements with several drugs, the degree of their improvement is typically modest, with marked residual deficits remaining, and at present no drug is satisfactory for this condition (Green, 1988).

In evaluating research, diagnostic criteria and the diagnostic heterogeneity/homogeneity of the sample, and both the severity of the patients included and the clinical setting in which the drug was given must be evaluated. Thus until the formalization by DSM-III (1980) of diagnostic distinctions between schizophrenia with childhood onset and autistic disorder (or their equivalents), both were subsumed under the diagnosis schizophrenia, childhood type, and many studies included diagnostically heterogeneous samples or the composition of the sample cannot be determined, rendering interpretation of the studies difficult or impossible (Campbell & Green, 1985).

Gadow and Poling (1988) provide another relevant example. They noted that stimulant medication is not commonly prescribed for the mentally retarded in residential facilities where most of the residents are usually severely or profoundly retarded. They pointed out that some reviews of the use of stimulants in the mentally retarded falling into these diagnostic categories suggested that stimulants might not be useful in treating behavior disorders in the retarded and could even exacerbate attentional deficit in these patients. Gadow and Poling (1988) noted that the large majority of mentally retarded individuals are not in institutions and that they are prescribed stimulants for management of disturbed behavior, particularly hyperactivity, much more frequently and with more favorable results than one might expect from reading the literature. In fact, these authors concluded that stimulants were highly effective in diminishing conduct problems and hyperactivity for some mentally retarded individuals, whatever their IQs.

As psychiatric nosology and diagnosis become more refined and the etiopathogeneses of more homogeneous subgroups are delineated, increasingly more focused research may be undertaken, and more specific and rational psychopharmacology will inevitably follow.

SPECIFIC DRUG TREATMENTS

In Part II of this book, psychopharmacological agents will be organized and discussed by class rather than according to the psychiatric diagnoses for which they are treatments. The rationale for this is related to several of the issues discussed in the first part of the book. At the present time most diagnoses are based on phenomenology, that is, constellations of clinical symptoms, rather than any basic understanding of the etiopathogenesis of the condition, and a given drug may be used to treat several psychiatric diagnoses. Hence repetition of facts under each diagnostic category and extensive cross-referencing are avoided.

Each class of drugs will be introduced with some general comments, including indications for use, contraindications, interactions with other drugs, and the most common untoward effects. The basic pharmacokinetics, including approximations of time of peak serum levels and the drug's serum half-life, major metabolites, and excretion, will be discussed. Unless otherwise noted, all dosage recommendations are for oral administration.

Specific drugs of each class will be reviewed individually; standard, FDA-approved treatments will be discussed first. Some treatments not approved for advertising by the FDA but reported to be efficacious in the literature and used clinically by some practitioners will be discussed as well. It is recommended that these drugs be used conservatively—that is, by experienced physicians and primarily after standard treatment regimens have proven unsuccessful. Likewise, a few drugs that have been investigated or are currently under investigation under research protocols and that seem to have potential therapeutic efficacy will also be reviewed; they should be used even more cautiously, if at all, in clinical practice.

Most of the studies cited herein either illustrate a particular point or provide the reader with some of the evidence, not readily accessible elsewhere, for using nonstandard treatments. This evidence ranges from reasonably convincing to merely suggesting a possible alternative for a seriously disturbed patient who has not responded satisfactorily to any standard, approved treatment. Excellent and extensive literature reviews of the standard psychopharmacological treatments discussed below are readily accessible in the additional readings given above.

Although always important, informed consent, preferably written, is particularly important if FDA-approved drugs are used for nonapproved indications. If standard approved treatments for a seriously disabling disorder have been tried with little or no success, a clinical trial of a nonapproved or even an investigational medication is much more easily justified. The physician has the responsibility to become thoroughly familiar with the official package labeling information provided by the manufacturer of the drug or the relevant entry in the latest edition and supplements of the PDR (1990) prior to prescribing any drug.

Table II.1 lists the most common psychiatric diagnoses in

Table II.1.
Diagnoses in Childhood and Adolescence for Which
Pharmacotherapy May Be Therapeutically Indicated

DSM-III-R Diagnosis	Medication
Mental retardation (with severe behavioral disorder and/or self-injurious behavior)	Thioridazine (p. 93) Chlorpromazine (pp. 92–93) Haloperidol (p. 96) Lithium (p. 155) (?) Propranolol (p. 180) (?) Naltrexone (p. 178)
Pervasive developmental disorders	Haloperidol (p. 98) (?) Fluphenazine (p. 102) (?) Naltrexone (p. 179) (?) Fenfluramine (p. 77)
Attention deficit hyperactivity disorder	Stimulants (p. 61) Tricyclics (p. 118, 126) Antipsychotics (p. 78) (?) Clonidine (p. 185) (?) Clomipramine (p. 132) (?) MAOIs (p. 136) (?) Bupropion (p. 141)
Conduct disorder (severe, aggressive)	Antipsychotics (p. 79) Haloperidol (p. 99) Lithium (p. 155) (?) Propranolol (p. 181) (?) Carbamazepine (p. 174)
Separation anxiety disorder	Imipramine (p. 119) (?) Chlordiazepoxide (p. 162)
Overanxious disorder	(?) Benzodiazepines (p. 157) Diphenhydramine (p. 171)
Tourette's disorder	Haloperidol (p. 97) Pimozide (p. 103) Clonidine (p. 188)
Functional encopresis	(?) Lithium (p. 156)
Functional enuresis	Imipramine (p. 113) (?) Benzodiazepines (p. 165) (?) Carbamazepine (p. 176) (?) Amphetamines (p. 53) (?) Clomipramine (p. 133)
Schizophrenia	Antipsychotics (p. 78)
Mania (acute and maintenance)	Lithium (p. 151) Antipsychotics (p. 78)
Major depression	Antidepressants (pp. 115, 120) (?) Lithium for Prophylaxis (p. 153) (?) Fluoxetine (p. 139) (?) Clomipramine (p. 133)
Obsessive-compulsive disorder	Clomipramine (p. 131) (?) Fluoxetine (p. 139)

(continued)

Table II.1. continued
Diagnoses in Childhood and Adolescence for Which
Pharmacotherapy May Be Therapeutically Indicated

DSM-III-R Diagnosis	Medication
Posttraumatic stress disorder (acute)	(?) Propranolol (p. 183)
Sleep disorders	
Insomnia disorder	Benzodiazepines (p. 157)
	Diphenhydramine (p. 171)
	Hydroxyzine (p. 172)
Sleep-wake schedule disorder	Benzodiazepines (p. 157)
	Diphenhydramine (p. 171)
	Hydroxyzine (p. 172)
Sleep terror disorder	Benzodiazepines (p. 166)
	(?) Imipramine (p. 120)
	(?) Carbamazepine (p. 175)
Sleepwalking disorder	Benzodiazepines (p. 166)
	(?) Imipramine (p. 120)
Intermittent explosive disorder	(?) Propranolol (p. 181)

children and younger adolescents for which psychopharmacotherapy may be therapeutically indicated and the drugs used
most frequently in treating that disorder. Where a specific drug or
class of drugs is generally preferred for a particular condition, an
attempt has been made to rank them in order of usual preference.

3

Sympathomimetic Amines and Central Nervous System Stimulants

INTRODUCTION

These drugs, commonly referred to as stimulants, are the drugs of choice for treating attention deficit hyperactivity disorder (ADHD). Bradley's 1937 report on the use of racemic amphetamine sulfate (Benzedrine) in behaviorally disordered children is usually cited as the beginning of child psychopharmacology as a discipline. Since this initial report, more research has been published on the stimulants and ADHD than on any other childhood disorder. Double-blind placebo-controlled studies have found consistently that stimulants are significantly superior to placebo in improving attention span and in decreasing hyperactivity and impulsivity. Although most of these studies have been done in children, two recent double-blind studies confirm the clinical efficacy of methylphenidate in treating adolescents diagnosed with attention deficit disorder (ADD) who also had had ADD as children (Klorman et al., 1988b).

Several reports in the more recent literature have found that methylphenidate also improved academic performance and peer interactions (see, e.g., Pelham et al., 1985, 1987). Whalen and her colleagues (1987) administered to 24 children between 6 and 11 years of age who were diagnosed with ADD or ADDH either placebo, 0.3 mg/kg methylphenidate daily, or 0.6 mg/kg methylphenidate daily, in a random order so that all children received each dosage level for a total of 4 days. The authors reported that all children showed decrements in negative social behaviors when rated during relatively unstructured outdoor activities at the 0.3 mg/kg level, compared to placebo. The youngest 12 children showed further improvement in social behavior at the higher dose level, but the older children showed no further improvement.

ADHD and conduct disorder may frequently coexist; in fact, DSM-III-R (APA, 1987) notes that if either diagnosis is present, the other diagnosis is commonly found as well. Psychostimulants also reduce some forms of aggression present in children diagnosed with attention deficit disorder with hyperactivity (ADDH) (Allen et al., 1975; Klorman et al., 1988b). Amery et al. (1984) compared dextroamphetamine and placebo in 10 boys diagnosed with ADDH with a mean age of 9.6 ± 1.6 years. Dextroamphetamine was administered in doses of 15 to 30 mg/day. The authors reported that scores on the Thematic Apperception Test Hostility Scale, the Holtzman Inkblot Test Hostility Scale, and observations for overt aggression in a laboratory free play situation were reduced significantly ($P < .05$) during a 2-week period on dextroamphetamine, compared to a similar period on placebo. These data are important, as ADHD and conduct disorder frequently coexist, and stimulants are often not considered in treating children whose conduct disorders are the primary consideration.

About 75% of ADHD children treated with stimulants will show favorable responses. Among these favorable responses, there will be a spectrum; some children will respond extremely well, others will benefit but to a lesser degree. Also, some children with ADHD (or an earlier equivalent diagnosis) will respond unfavorably to one stimulant drug but favorably to another. For example, Arnold et al. (1976) conducted a double-blind cross-over study of D-amphetamine, L-amphetamine, and placebo in 31 children with minimal brain dysfunction (MBD). Both isomers were statistically superior to placebo and did not differ significantly from each other. Interestingly, of the 25 children with positive responses, 17 responded well to both isomers, 5 responded favorably only to the D-isomer, and 3 responded favorably only to the L-isomer (Arnold et al., 1976).

Wender (1988) notes that the development of tolerance to the therapeutic effects of stimulant medication is unusual and that when it occurs, it progresses gradually over a period of a year or two. If this occurs, a trial of another stimulant is suggested, as complete cross-tolerance among the stimulants does not occur (Wender, 1988).

Gadow and Poling (1988) have reviewed the literature on the use of stimulants in the mentally retarded and concluded that stimulants are highly effective in reducing symptoms of hyperactivity and conduct disorder in some individuals whatever the degree of their retardation.

Normal prepubertal boys and college-age men reacted similarly to patients diagnosed with ADHD when given single doses of dextroamphetamine; they exhibited decreased motor activity and generally improved attentional performance (Rapoport et al., 1978a, 1980a). Hence earlier teachings that stimulants have a paradoxical effect in hyperactive children are incorrect, and a positive response to stimulant medication cannot be used to validate the diagnosis of ADHD.

PHARMACOKINETICS OF STIMULANTS

The stimulants undergo some metabolism in the liver and are primarily excreted by the kidneys. Table 3.1 gives the site of metabolism, main metabolic products, time of peak plasma levels, serum half-lives, and routes of excretion for the stimulants commonly used in child and adolescent psychiatry.

CONTRAINDICATIONS FOR STIMULANT ADMINISTRATION

Known hypersensitivity to the medication is an absolute contraindication.

Stimulants may cause stereotypies, tics, and psychosis *de novo* in sensitive individuals or if given in high enough doses. Stimulants are relatively contraindicated in children and adolescents with a history of schizophrenia or other psychosis, pervasive developmental disorders, or borderline personality organization, as they appear to worsen these conditions in many cases. There is considerable controversy over whether they should be given to children and adolescents with Tourette's disorder, a tic disorder, or a family history of such disorders. Their use in pervasive developmental disorders and in Tourette's disorder or with tic disorders is discussed in greater detail below.

Stimulants may aggravate symptoms of marked anxiety, tension, and agitation and are contraindicated when these symptoms are prominent (manufacturer's package insert).

Table 3.1.
Some Pharmacokinetic Properties of Stimulant Drugs

Drug	Principal Metabolite(s)	Peak Serum Levels	Serum Half-Life	Principal Route(s) of Excretion
Methylphenidate (Ritalin)	Liver → 75% ritalinic acid, which is pharmacologically inactive	1.9 hr (range, 0.3–4.4 hr); Ritalin S-R, 4.7 hr (range, 1.3–8.2 hr)	2–2½ hr	Kidney excretes 70%–80% primarily as ritalinic acid, in 24 hr
Dextroamphetamine sulfate (Dexedrine)	Liver → P-hydroxylation, N-demethylation, deamination, and conjugation	2 hours for tablet; 8–10 hr for spansule	6–8 hr in children, 10–12 hr in adults	May be excreted unchanged by kidney. Amount varies according to urinary pH—from 2% to 3% in very alkaline urine to 80% in acidic urine.
Magnesium pemoline (Cylert)	Liver → pemoline conjugates: pemoline dione, mandelic acid, and other products	2–4 hr	8–12 hr	Kidney excretes about 40%–50% unchanged, plus about 25%–40% as products of liver metabolism.

Stimulants have a potential to be abused. They should not be prescribed to patients who have a history of drug abuse or where there is a likelihood family members or friends would abuse the medication.

Magnesium pemoline should not be administered to patients with impaired liver function or to those with known hypersensitivity to it.

INTERACTIONS OF STIMULANTS WITH OTHER DRUGS

Stimulants should not be administered with monoamine oxidase inhibitors (MAOIs) or until a period of at least 14 days has elapsed since MAOIs were ingested, to avoid possible hypertensive crises.

In combination with tricyclic antidepressants, the actions of both may be enhanced.

Stimulants potentiate sympathomimetic drugs (including street amphetamines and cocaine) and may counteract the sedative effect of antihistamines and benzodiazepines.

Lithium may inhibit the stimulatory effects of amphetamines.

Amphetamines may act synergistically with phenytoin or phenobarbital to increase anticonvulsant activity.

Many other drug interactions, which are less likely to be encountered in child and adolescent psychiatry, may occur.

UNTOWARD EFFECTS OF STIMULANTS

There is some evidence that overall, the untoward effects of methylphenidate occur less frequently and with less severity than those from dextroamphetamine (Conners, 1971; Gross & Wilson, 1974). Gross and Wilson (1974) noted that side effects were infrequently severe enough to make immediate discontinuation of medication necessary—1.1% of 377 patients for methylphenidate, and 4.3% of 371 patients for dextroamphetamine.

The most frequent and troublesome immediate untoward effects include insomnia, anorexia, nausea, abdominal pain or cramps, headache, thirst, vomiting, lability of mood, irritability, sadness, weepiness, tachycardia, and blood pressure changes. Many of these symptoms diminish over a period of up to a few weeks, although the cardiovascular changes may persist.

Since 1972 disturbances in growth—decrements in both height and weight percentiles—have been reported for both methylphenidate and dextroamphetamine, and the long-term untoward consequences of these effects have been of particular concern (Safer et al., 1972). There has been controversy about how significant these changes are. Mattes and Gittelman (1983) reported significant decreases in height and weight percentiles over a 4-year period. A recently published controlled study found a significant reduction in growth velocity during the period of time that stimulants are actively administered (Klein et al., 1988). Despite this adverse effect on growth during the active treatment phase, it appears that an accelerated rate of growth or growth rebound occurs once the stimulant is discontinued and that there is usually no significant compromise of ultimate height attained (Klein & Mannuzza, 1988). It seems likely, however, that some children are at greater risk for growth suppression than others, and careful serial heights and weights of any child receiving stimulant medication should be plotted on a growth chart (e.g., the National Center for Health Statistics Growth Chart) (Hamill et al., 1976) for any child receiving stimulants.

Vincent et al. (1990) reported no significant deviations from expected height and weight growth velocities in 31 adolescents diagnosed with ADHD who had received methylphenidate continuously for a minimum of 6 months to a maximum of 6 years after their twelfth birthdays. Mean age at beginning the study was 12.9 ± 0.8 years. The mean daily dose was 34 ± 14 mg or 0.75 ± 0.29 mg/kg and did not differ significantly with age or sex. The results suggested that early adolescent growth is not significantly adversely affected by methylphenidate.

A few children treated with stimulants may develop a clinical picture resembling schizophrenia. This most frequently occurs when untoward effects such as disorganization are misinterpreted as a worsening of presenting symptoms and the dosage is further increased until prominent psychotomimetic effects occur. This may also occur when stimulants are administered to children with borderline personality disorders or schizophrenia, conditions in which stimulants are usually contraindicated. In most such cases, the psychotic symptomatology improves rapidly following discontinuation of the drug (Green, 1989).

Some parents express concern that treatment with stimulants will predispose their child to later drug abuse or addiction. Most available evidence indicates that this is not the case. Although drug abuse itself is of major concern in our culture, children who have been treated for their ADHD with stimulants appear to be at no greater risk than controls for drug or alcohol abuse as teenagers and adults (Weiss & Hechtman, 1986).

Rebound Effects of Stimulants

Rebound effects may occur beginning about 5 hours after the last dose of methylphenidate. Behavioral symptoms of rebound are often identical to those of the ADHD being treated and, in some cases, may even exceed baseline levels prior to administration of stimulants.

Rapoport and her colleagues reported that normal children who were administered dextroamphetamine experienced behavioral rebound about 5 hours after a single acute dose. Symptoms included excitability, talkativeness, overactivity, insomnia, stomachaches, and mild nausea (Rapoport et al., 1978a).

STIMULANTS' RELATIONSHIP TO TICS AND TOURETTE'S DISORDER

Stimulants can exacerbate existing tics and precipitate tics and stereotypies *de novo.* There is disagreement among experts as to whether stimulants should be given to persons with tics, Tourette's disorder, or a family history of either.

In a study of 1520 children diagnosed with ADDH and treated with methylphenidate, Denckla et al. (1976) reported that existing tics were exacerbated in 6 cases (0.39%) and tics developed *de novo* in 14 cases (0.92%). Following the discontinuation of methylphenidate, all the 6 tics that had worsened returned to their premedication intensity, and 13 of the 14 new tics completely remitted.

Shapiro and Shapiro (1981) reviewed the relationship between treating ADDH with stimulants and the precipitation or exacerbation of tics and Tourette's syndrome (TS). They also noted that they had treated 42 patients for symptoms of both MBD and TS with a combination of methylphenidate and haloperidol. Dosage of methylphenidate ranged from 5 to 60 mg/day and was individually titrated for each patient. The authors also used methylphenidate (dose range 5 to 40 mg/day) in 62 additional patients with TS to counteract untoward effects of haloperidol, such as sedation, amotivation, dysphoria, cognitive impairment, and dullness. Shapiro and Shapiro (1981) concluded that the evidence suggests that stimulants do not cause or provoke TS, although high doses of stimulants can cause or exacerbate tics in predisposed patients. Clinically they noted that tics seemed less likely to be exacerbated by stimulants in patients who were also taking haloperidol for TS; when tics did increase in intensity, this remitted within 3 to 6 hours, the approximate duration of the usual clinical effects of methylphenidate.

Lowe et al. (1982) reported on a series of 15 patients diagnosed with ADDH who were treated with stimulant medications, including methylphenidate, dextroamphetamine, and pemoline, who subsequently had tics develop *de novo*, or existing tics worsen, sometimes into full-blown cases of Tourette's disorder. Nine subjects had existing tics; 8 had family histories of tics or Tourette's disorder. Twelve of the 15 cases eventually required medication for control of the tics. The authors considered the presence of Tourette's disorder or tics to be a contraindication to stimulant medication and that stimulants should be used with much caution in the presence of a family history of tics or Tourette's disorder. They also considered the development of tics following treatment with stimulants sufficient reason to discontinue use of stimulant medication.

Lowe et al. (1982) noted that the early clinical signs of Tourette's disorder may be difficult to differentiate from attention deficit disorder with hyperactivity (ADDH). Shapiro and Shapiro (1981) noted that about 57% of children with tic and Tourette's syndromes (TTS) had concomitant minimal brain dysfunction (MBD), although most children with MBD do not develop TTS. Comings and Comings (1984) investigated the relationship between Tourette's syndrome (TS) and ADDH. They found ADDH was present in 62% of 140 males under age 21 years diagnosed with TS. A study of their family pedigrees suggested that the TS gene could be expressed as ADDH but without tics. The authors felt their data implied that patients diagnosed ADDH and treated with stimulants who subsequently developed tics had ADDH as a result of the TS gene and probably would have developed tics or TS even if they had not been treated with stimulant medication.

At the present time, a conservative approach would consider the stimulants relatively or absolutely contraindicated in treating children and adolescents with tics or Tourette's syndrome, and a reason for caution in the presence of family history of such. In fact, one manufacturer of methylphenidate states that it is contraindicated in patients with motor tics or with a family history or diagnosis of Tourette's syndrome.

THE STIMULANT DRUGS APPROVED FOR USE IN CHILD AND ADOLESCENT PSYCHIATRY

The stimulants are the most frequently prescribed psychiatric drugs during childhood. In 1977 more that half a million children were being treated with methylphenidate in the United States alone (Sprague & Sleator, 1977). Because methylphenidate is the most commonly prescribed drug for ADHD, it will be used to illustrate the use of the stimulants, despite its having appeared on the scene considerably later than dextroamphetamine sulfate.

Methylphenidate (Ritalin)

Indications in Child and Adolescent Psychiatry
FDA approved for treating attention deficit hyperactivity disorder (ADHD) and narcolepsy.

Dosage Schedule for Treating ADHD
- Children under 6 years old: Not approved for use.
- Persons 6 years of age and over: Start with 5 mg once or twice daily and raise dose gradually 5 to 10 mg/week. Maximum recommended daily dosage is 60 mg.
- The usual optimal dose of methylphenidate falls between 0.3 and 0.7 mg/kg/dose administered two to three times daily (total daily dose of 0.9 to 2.1 mg/kg/day) (Duncan, 1990).

Dose Forms Available
- Tablets: 5 mg, 10 mg, 20 mg
- Sustained release tablets (Ritalin-SR): 20 mg

Pharmacokinetics of Methylphenidate

Administration of methylphenidate with meals does not appear to adversely affect its absorption or pharmacokinetics and may diminish problems with appetite suppression (Patrick et al., 1987).

An improvement of target symptoms can be seen in as few as 20 minutes after a therapeutically effective dose is given (Zametkin et al., 1985). Peak blood levels occur between 1 to 2$\frac{1}{2}$ hours after administration (Gualtieri et al., 1982), and the serum half-life is about 2$\frac{1}{2}$ hours (Winsberg et al., 1982). Patrick et al. (1987) have reviewed the pharmacokinetics of methylphenidate in detail. The major metabolite produced in the liver is ritalinic acid, which is pharmacologically inactive. Between 70% and 80% of the radioactivity of radiolabeled methylphenidate, over 75% of which is ritalinic acid, is recovered in the urine within 24 hours.

Because of these pharmacokinetics, the most frequent times to administer methylphenidate to children and adolescents are before leaving for school and during the lunch hour. This dosage schedule usually ensures adequate serum levels during school hours, which is the foremost consideration for most students.

Sustained release tablets make once-daily dosage possible for some children. However, there is some evidence that the clinical efficacy of sustained release methylphenidate is delayed about an hour and that it is not as effective as the standard form. Pelham and his colleagues (1987) found significant differences in efficacy between standard methylphenidate and sustained release methylphenidate on several important measures of disruptive behavior in two studies of a total of 22 boys with ADHD. These authors felt that if once-daily dosage was a necessity, that slow-release dextroamphetamine or magnesium pemoline would often be preferable to sustained release methylphenidate. Birmaher et al. (1989) noted that the maximum serum level takes longer to develop when sustained release tablets are administered and that peak serum levels are lower than for an equivalent dose of standard methylphenidate. These authors suggested that the relative inefficacy of sustained release methylphenidate could be because of differences in pharmacokinetics or absorption, or tachyphylaxis.

Untoward Effects and Adjustment of Methylphenidate Dose Schedule

Children who develop significant behavioral or attentional difficulties in the late afternoon or early evening may do so because of a return to baseline behavior as serum levels decline into subtherapeutic levels and/or because of a rebound effect as the drug wears off (Rapoport et al., 1978a). A third dose of medication given in the afternoon may be helpful for some such children. A recent study, however, suggests that psychostimulant rebound effects are not clinically significant for the large majority of children (Johnston et al., 1988).

Insomnia may also occur. It is clinically important to distinguish those children whose insomnia is an untoward effect of the drug from those children whose insomnia may be due to the recurrence of behavioral difficulties as the medication effect subsides and/or to a rebound effect. For the first group of children, a reduction in milligram dosage of the last dose of the day may be necessary. For the latter group, an evening dose or a dose about an hour before bedtime may be helpful. Chatoor et al. (1983) prescribed late afternoon or evening dextroamphetamine sustained release capsules to seven children who had strong rebound effects as their medication wore off and who developed marked behavioral problems and difficulty settling down and sleeping at bedtime. Parents reported significant behavioral improvement and markedly less bedtime oppositional behavior and increased ease in falling asleep. The authors compared sleep EEGs in seven children recorded during periods on dextroamphetamine sustained release capsules and on placebo. Compared to placebo, dextroamphetamine tended to delay onset of sleep slightly, significantly increased rapid eye movement (REM) latency (time to first REM period), and significantly decreased REM time (by about 14%) and the number of REM periods. Length of stage 1 and stage 2 sleep was significantly increased, and sleep efficiency (amount of time asleep during recording) decreased. Reduction in sleep efficiency was only 5%, which seemed minor compared to the significant behavioral improvement that occurred (Chatoor et al., 1983).

There is some evidence that methylphenidate may lower the convulsive threshold (manufacturer's package insert). McBride et al. (1986), however, found only a single case report in the literature in which a child who was previously seizure free had a seizure soon after treatment with methylphenidate was begun. The authors treated 23 children and adolescents aged 4 years to 15 years and diagnosed with ADD who had seizure disorders of various types (N = 20) or epileptiform EEG abnormalities (N = 3) with methylphenidate. Fifteen of the children with documented seizure disorder received concomitant antiepileptic drugs. Individual doses of 0.33 mg/kg (± 0.13 mg/kg) were administered with total daily doses of 0.63 mg/kg (± 0.25 mg/kg) for 3 months up to 4 years' duration. The authors found no evidence of increased frequency of seizures following methylphenidate treatment in 16 children with active seizure disorders or 4 children who had had active seizure disorders but who had been seizure free and off antiepileptic drugs for from 2 months to 2 years. The three children with epileptiform abnormalities also developed no seizures during the period they received methylphenidate. This evidence suggests that methylphenidate may not lower the seizure threshold to a clinically significant degree at usual therapeutic doses and that the presence of a seizure disorder in a child or adolescent with ADHD is not a contraindication for a trial of methylphenidate (McBride et al., 1986). Crumrine et al. (1987) also reported that they had administered methylphenidate 0.3 mg/kg twice daily to 9 males 6.1 years to 10.1 years of age who had diagnoses of AHDH and seizure disorder. The boys had been previously stabilized on anticonvulsant medication and experienced no seizures or changes in EEG background patterns or epileptiform activity during 4-week randomized double-blind cross-over trials of methylphenidate or placebo. Subjects improved significantly on the hyperactivity, inattention, and hyperactivity index factors on the Conners Teacher Questionnaire (Crumrine et al., 1987).

These reports suggest that when clinically indicated, it is not unreasonable to undertake a trial of methylphenidate in children and adolescents with coexisting seizure disorders and ADHD. Clearly, frequency of seizures should be carefully monitored, and if their frequency increases or seizures develop de novo, the clinician may discontinue methylphenidate.

Swanson et al. (1986) reported on six children who developed behavioral and cognitive tolerance to their usual doses of methylphenidate during long-term treatment. To maintain satisfactory clinical response, their pediatricians had to titrate their total daily doses to levels of 120 mg to 300 mg administered in as many as five individual doses of 40 mg to 60 mg. These children performed a cognitive task better at their usual high dose (average, 60 mg three times daily) than at a lower dose (average, 30 mg three times daily), confirming cognitive tolerance. Overall, these children had high serum levels compatible with the high doses, suggesting that neither metabolic tolerance nor differential absorption was responsible for the behavioral tolerance.

Garfinkel et al. (1983) compared efficacy of methylphenidate with placebo, desipramine, and clomipramine in a double-blind cross-over study of 12 males (mean age, 7.3 years; range, 5.9 to 11.6 years) diagnosed with ADD who required day hospital or inpatient hospitalization for the severity of their impulsivity, inattention, and aggressiveness. Methylphenidate was significantly better in improving symptoms on the Conners Scale as rated by teachers ($P < .005$) and program child care workers ($P < .001$).

Investigational Reports of Interest

Methylphenidate has been investigated in the treatment of hyperactive children with autistic disorder. Although most of the earlier literature states that stimulants are contraindicated for autistic children and cause a worsening in behavior and/or stereo-typies, several recent studies have reported that methylphenidate is effective in treating some children with autistic disorder who also exhibit such symptoms as hyperactivity, impulsivity, short attention spans, and aggression. Strayhorn et al. (1988) reported on two autistic children, a 6-year-old autistic boy given meth-ylphenidate in a randomized trial with either placebo or meth-ylphenidate given each day, and a preschool child treated openly with methylphenidate. The former child was reported to show improvement in attention and activity levels, less destructive behavior, and a decrease in stereotyped movements, but sadness and temper tantrums significantly worsened. The preschooler was said to have had similar results.

Birmaher et al. (1988) treated nine hyperactive autistic chil-dren aged 4 years to 16 years with 10 to 50 mg/day of methylpheni-date. Eight of the children improved on all rating scales; the oldest child improved on all scales except the one measuring behavior in school.

On the other hand, Realmuto et al. (1989), who treated two 9-year-old autistic boys with 10 mg of methylphenidate adminis-tered twice daily, found that one became fearful and unable to separate from significant adults, had a worsening of his hyperac-tivity, and developed a rapid pulse, while the second youngster's baseline behaviors did not significantly change, although he de-veloped mild anorexia.

Until additional research with larger samples of autistic chil-dren clarifies these studies, the use of methylphenidate in treating autistic children or hyperactive subgroups of them must be re-garded as investigational.

Dextroamphetamine Sulfate (Dexedrine)

Indications in Child and Adolescent Psychiatry
FDA approved for treating attention deficit disorder with hyper-activity (ADDH), narcolepsy, and exogenous obesity. (ADDH is a DSM-III [1980] diagnosis that, in large part, corresponds to the DSM-III-R [1987] diagnosis ADHD; technically, as late as 1990 the FDA approval for advertising is still for treatment of ADDH; however, for purposes of medication and dosage, these diagnoses are essentially equivalent.)

Dosage Schedule for Treating ADDH/ADHD
- Children under 3 years of age: Not approved for use.
- Children 3 through 5 years: Begin with 2.5 mg daily; raise by 2.5-mg increments once or twice weekly; titrate for optimal dose.
- Patients 6 years and over: Begin with 5 mg daily; raise by 5-mg increments once or twice weekly; usual maximum dose is less than 40 mg/day.
- The usual optimal daily dose falls between 0.15 and 0.5 mg/kg/dose, administered two to three times daily (total daily dose range, 0.30 to 1.5 mg/kg/day) (Duncan, 1990).

Dose Forms Available
- Elixir: 5 mg/5 ml
- Tablets: 5 mg
- Sustained release capsules (Spansules): 5 mg, 10 mg, 15 mg

Dextroamphetamine in the Treatment of ADDH/ADHD

Dextroamphetamine sulfate is the only amphetamine currently used with any frequency to treat ADHD and is the only stimulant currently in use that is approved by the FDA for administration to children as young as 3 years of age. Hence it is officially the drug of choice for children up to age 6 years, when most clinicians appear to prefer methylphenidate. In addition, if methylphenidate does not provide satisfactory benefit in controlling symptoms of ADHD, it is recommended that dextroamphetamine and/or pemoline be tried before moving on to another class of drugs.

Amphetamines may obtund the maximal electroshock seizure discharge and have been reported to prevent typical 3-per-second spike-and-dome petit mal seizures and to abolish the abnormal EEG pattern in some children (Weiner, 1980). Dextroamphetamine may thus be the stimulant of choice for individuals who have seizures or who are at risk for developing them, although, as noted above, methylphenidate does not appear to increase the frequency of seizures or their development de novo when used in usual therapeutic doses.

Investigational Report of Interest

Geller et al. (1981) reported that dextroamphetamine administered to two children with pervasive developmental disorder and ADDH improved their attention spans with no significant worsening of behavior.

Magnesium Pemoline (Cylert)

Indications in Child and Adolescent Psychiatry
   FDA approved for the treatment of attention deficit disorder with hyperactivity (ADDH). (ADDH is a DSM-III [1980] diagnosis that, in large part, corresponds to the DSM-III-R [1987] diagnosis ADHD; technically, as late as 1990 the FDA approval for advertising is still for treatment of ADDH; however, for purposes of medication and dosage, these diagnoses are essentially equivalent.)

Dosage Schedule for Treating ADDH/ADHD
* Children under age 6 years: Not recommended for use.
* Persons 6 years of age and over: The initial recommended daily dose of pemoline is 37.5 mg. This may be increased weekly by 18.75 mg until satisfactory clinical benefit occurs, untoward effects prevent further increase, or the maximum daily dose of 112.5 mg is reached.

Dose Forms Available
* Tablets: 18.75 mg, 37.5 mg, 75 mg

Magnesium Pemoline in the Treatment of ADHD

Magnesium pemoline elicits central nervous system changes that are similar to those of methylphenidate and amphetamines, but it is structurally dissimilar to those drugs and has minimal sympathomimetic effects. Its serum half-life is approximately 12 hours. About 90% of an oral dose of magnesium pemoline is excreted by the kidneys; this consists of unmetabolized magnesium pemoline (between 40% and 50%) and a remainder comprised of metabolic products of magnesium pemoline that were formed in the liver.

Sallee et al. (1985) reported a 200% variability in pemoline's bioavailability, a 300% variation in total body clearance of pemoline, and a 600% variation in elimination half-time among 7 prepubescent hyperactive boys. They also suggested there may be a relatively narrow therapeutic margin and noted that choreiform movements occur frequently after an acute dose of 2 mg/kg/day of magnesium pemoline.

Advantages of pemoline over the sympathomimetic amines thus include minimal untoward cardiovascular effects; a longer serum half-life, permitting a single morning dose daily (if sustained release forms of the other stimulants are not available to the patient); and probably having a less intense rebound effect than methylphenidate and dextroamphetamine. The disadvantages of pemoline are that its clinical effect is not as great as that of dextroamphetamine and methylphenidate, and improvement occurs gradually rather than promptly (Conners et al., 1972). If the manufacturer's recommended titration regimen is followed, significant clinical benefit from pemoline is often apparent only after 3 to 4 weeks. Another concern is hepatotoxicity. Elevated liver enzymes occur in a small percentage, perhaps 1% to 3%, of children treated with magnesium pemoline; these abnormalities appear to be reversible following drug withdrawal, but it is essential to monitor liver function regularly with liver function tests throughout the duration of therapy (PDR, 1990).

Sallee et al. (1985, 1989) reported that acute exposure to a single 2 mg/kg dose of pemoline resulted in abnormal involuntary movements including buccal-lingual chewing and choreoathetoid movements of the face, extremities, and trunk in 25% (5 of 20) of severely hyperactive 6- to 12-year-old boys. The movements occurred at peak plasma pemoline concentration or immediately thereafter and lasted for up to 8 hours but persisted with repeated doses in only one subject. This subject and three additional patients also developed choreiform movements after receiving pemoline for a minimum of 3 weeks (3 patients received 2 mg/kg/day of pemoline, and 1 patient received 1.5 mg/kg/day of pemoline and 10 mg/day of imipramine). The authors noted that the low frequency of choreiform movements reported during the clinical use of pemoline may result from the gradual titration of pemoline. These data would suggest that the clinician should not increase the dosage of pemoline more rapidly than recommended.

Another important observation was that improvement in focusing attention occurred within 2 to 3 hours after the dose of pemoline in the acute trial, as opposed to the typically much longer lag period for significant clinical improvement when pemoline is prescribed as recommended (Sallee et al., 1989).

Fenfluramine (Pondimin)

Indications for Use in Child and Adolescent Psychiatry
Fenfluramine, a sympathomimetic amine with antiserotonergic properties, is approved by the FDA only as a short-term adjunct to the treatment of exogenous obesity in persons 12 years of age or older.

Investigational Reports of Interest

Fenfluramine has been investigated in the treatment of ADDH and autistic disorder. Clinically fenfluramine was not efficacious, and it had no beneficial effects on motor activity or behavioral ratings in the treatment of ADDH (Donnelly et al., 1989). The rationale for fenfluramine's investigational use in the treatment of autistic disorder was based on the fact that it decreases serotonin levels, which have been found to be elevated in about 30% of mentally retarded and autistic children. Ritvo and his colleagues (Ritvo et al., 1983) reported favorable results in a study of 14 autistic children, which stimulated several other investigators to study this drug.

A 1988 review of published studies of fenfluramine use with autistic children suggested that a subgroup of autistic children with the highest IQ levels and the lowest serotonin values and who had hyperactivity and motor stereotypies improved somewhat with the drug (Verglas et al., 1988). On the other hand, a double-blind placebo-controlled study of 28 autistic children found that fenfluramine was not statistically superior to placebo and that it had a retarding effect on discrimination learning, and noted that no individual children had a strong, positive response to the drug (Campbell et al., 1988). Thus although initially there were some encouraging data, they have not been replicated. Further evaluation of the clinical efficacy and safety of fenfluramine must be undertaken and more positive results must be obtained before its use in autistic disorder can be regarded as other than investigational.

Caffeine

Caffeine is included here as there have been some suggestions that it may be useful in treating ADHD. Two reviews of the relevant literature concluded that caffeine is not a therapeutically useful drug in the treatment of ADHD (Klein, 1987; Klein et al., 1980).

4

Antipsychotic Drugs

INTRODUCTION

Although in adults these drugs, also commonly referred to as neuroleptics or major tranquilizers, are used primarily to treat psychoses, in children they have additionally been used to treat other common nonpsychotic psychiatric disorders. One reason for this seems to be that the antipsychotics won by default; they were among the earliest psychoactive drugs used in child psychiatry, and the competition hadn't arrived yet. In addition, the risk of untoward effects such as cognitive dulling and irreversible tardive dyskinesia had not been fully appreciated. As clinical and research experience in child psychopharmacology progresses and other drugs become available, however, the use of these drugs in children is becoming more circumscribed, and indications for their use in children are more and more closely approaching those for which they are prescribed in older adolescents and adults.

At the present time, antipsychotics are the drugs of first choice in childhood for schizophrenia and autistic disorder. There is, however, some evidence that antipsychotics are not as effective clinically in schizophrenia with childhood onset as in schizophrenia occurring in later adolescence and adulthood (Green et al., 1984). Meyers et al. (1980) noted that serum neuroleptic levels of 50 ng/ml of chlorpromazine equivalents correspond to the threshold for clinical response in adult schizophrenics and suggest that similar therapeutic serum levels are necessary in children. Because children may metabolize and excrete antipsychotics more efficiently than adults, determination of serum neuroleptic levels, if they are available, is recommended before a trial of an antipsychotic is deemed a failure.

Shapiro and Shapiro (1989) concluded that antipsychotics were also the drugs of choice for treating chronic motor or vocal tic disorder and Tourette's disorder when psychosocial, educational, or occupational functioning was so impaired that medication was required. Although antipsychotics are probably indicated in acute mania, paranoia, and schizoaffective disorder, these disorders are rarely diagnosed in childhood, and there is little information available on the use of antipsychotics to treat children with these diagnoses.

Antipsychotics are also clinically effective in severely aggressive, conduct-disordered children, and some are approved for use in such children. Lithium, however, is also effective in such children, perhaps more so when there is explosive affect present, and lithium has fewer clinically significant untoward effects than neuroleptics. Because lithium is still not approved for use for either children under 12 years of age or for this indication, and because of the necessity of monitoring serum lithium levels, most clinicians continue to use antipsychotics at the present time.

The use of antipsychotics in the mentally retarded continues to be controversial, but they are prescribed frequently, especially for institutionalized patients. Only three neuroleptics are recognized by the FDA as effective for the treatment of psychiatric disorders in the mentally retarded: thioridazine, chlorpromazine, and haloperidol (Gadow & Poling, 1988). In optimal doses antipsychotics are effective in decreasing irritability, sleep disturbances, hostility, agitation, and combativeness and may improve concentration and social behavior in agitated, severely retarded individuals (American Medical Association, 1986). Aman and Singh (1988) cautioned that the influential studies of the mentally retarded by Breuning, which showed significant detrimental effects resulting from antipsychotics, appear to have been fabricated.

Some antipsychotics (e.g., thioridazine) have been approved for treating children with symptoms such as excessive motor activity, impulsivity, difficulty sustaining attention, and poor frustration tolerance, which would be found in most children diagnosed with ADHD. Although antipsychotics improve some symptoms of children with ADHD (Gittelman-Klein et al., 1976), untoward effects such as cognitive dulling and the risk of tardive dyskinesia limit their clinical usefulness primarily to children who do not respond satisfactorily to stimulants or antidepressants.

In a randomized cross-over double-blind study, Weizman et

al. (1984) reported that the combination of propericiazine, a neuroleptic frequently prescribed by Israeli child psychiatrists, and a stimulant was statistically superior to placebo-stimulant treatment of 14 children diagnosed with ADDH who had experienced some, but not satisfactory, improvement with stimulant medication only. The authors noted that the combination of a stimulant and neuroleptics may be useful in some children who do not respond adequately to stimulants alone. They also noted that the purported therapeutic effects of stimulants are secondary to their increasing dopamine release, and that those of neuroleptics are secondary to their being dopamine blockers; the synergistic effect of the two agents suggests that more complicated mechanisms than simple dopamine release or blockade are involved (Weizman et al., 1984). Clinically this may be a potentially useful option for a small subgroup of children who do not respond adequately to stimulants or to tricyclics alone, as presumably the combination of stimulant and neuroleptic would achieve a satisfactory result that either would not be achieved by neuroleptic alone or would require higher doses of neuroleptics, which would carry an increased risk of untoward effects such as tardive dyskinesia and cognitive dulling.

PHARMACOKINETICS OF ANTIPSYCHOTICS

Rivera-Calimlim et al. (1979) reported plasma chlorpromazine levels in a total of 24 children aged 8 to 16 years who were treated with chlorpromazine for psychiatric disorders, including various psychoses, mental retardation with aggression, hyperactivity, self-injurious behavior, and mood disorders with anxiety. The authors reported wide interpatient variations in chlorpromazine plasma levels for a given dose; for example, 9 children receiving 0.8 to 2.9 mg/kg/day achieved mean plasma levels of 6.6 ng/ml, with a range from undetectable to 18 ng/ml. One child receiving 9.8 mg/kg showed only trace levels of plasma chlorpromazine. Children and adolescents had chlorpromazine plasma levels that were from 2 times to 3.5 times lower than those for adults, for a given dose per kilogram body weight. Clinical improvement in these children usually began when plasma chlorpromazine concentration was at least 30 ng/ml, and optimal levels ranged between 40 ng/ml and 80 ng/ml, as compared to adults treated with chlorpromazine, where suggested optimal plasma levels were higher, between 50 ng/ml and 300 ng/ml. A final clinically important observation was that plasma chlorpromazine levels declined over time in most patients who were on fixed doses (Rivera-Calimlim et al., 1979). It was suggested that one possible reason for this might be autoinduction of enzymes that metabolize chlorpromazine.

CONTRAINDICATIONS FOR ANTIPSYCHOTIC ADMINISTRATION

Known hypersensitivity to the drug and toxic central nervous system depression or comatose states are absolute contraindications. If a severe untoward effect develops (e.g., agranulocytosis, neuroleptic malignant syndrome, tardive dyskinesia, or a withdrawal dyskinesia), children and adolescents should be managed without antipsychotics if at all possible.

Neuroleptics may lower the seizure threshold; they should be used cautiously in patients with seizure disorders, and chlorpromazine probably should not be used in such patients.

INTERACTIONS OF ANTIPSYCHOTICS WITH OTHER DRUGS

The most frequent clinically important reactions are with other central nervous system depressants such as alcohol, sedatives and hypnotics, benzodiazepines, antihistamines, opiates, and barbiturates, where an additive central nervous system depressive effect occurs.

Antipsychotics also have varying degrees of anticholinergic effects. When combined with another anticholinergic (antiparkinsonian) agent, as when one is used prophylactically to prevent acute dyskinesia, pseudoparkinsonism, or akathisia, central nervous system symptoms of cholinergic blockade may result. These symptoms may include confusion, disorientation, delirium, hallucinations, and worsening of preexisting psychotic symptoms. Of clinical importance, this picture may be mistaken for inadequate treatment or worsening of the psychosis, rather than an untoward effect.

The combination of antipsychotics and lithium carbonate, particularly if high doses are used, may possibly lead to an increased incidence of central nervous system toxicity, including neuroleptic malignant syndrome.

Combined use with tricyclic antidepressants or monoamine oxidase inhibitors may increase plasma levels of antidepressants.

Neuroleptics may also have noteworthy interactions with many other medications.

UNTOWARD EFFECTS OF ANTIPSYCHOTICS

While antipsychotic drugs may have numerous serious untoward effects, those of greatest concern in children and adolescents are the effects of sedation on cognition and the extrapyramidal syndromes, in particular the possible development of irreversible tardive dyskinesia.

Agranulocytosis

Agranulocytosis has also been reported with antipsychotics. It usually occurs relatively early in treatment (e.g., for chlorpromazine usually between the 4th and 10th weeks). Parents and older patients should be warned to report indications of sudden infections, such as fever and sore throat, to the physician. White blood count should be determined immediately, and if it is significantly depressed, medication should be stopped and therapy instituted.

Untoward Cognitive Effects

Both high-potency and low-potency antipsychotics are effective when given in equivalent doses, but they differ in the frequency and severity of their untoward effects. Usually, the higher-potency antipsychotics cause less sedation, fewer autonomic side effects, and more extrapyramidal untoward effects, and the lower potency antipsychotics cause greater sedation, more autonomic side effects, and fewer extrapyramidal effects (Baldessarini, 1990). Because of the great importance of minimizing any cognitive dulling in schoolchildren and in the mentally retarded, whose cognition is already compromised, high-potency, less-sedative antipsychotics are often preferred. Over a period of days to weeks, however, considerable tolerance often develops to the sedative effects of high-dose, low-potency antipsychotics, and they are still useful when untoward effects are carefully monitored (Green, 1989).

Extrapyramidal Syndromes

Significant numbers of children and adolescents receiving antipsychotic medication develop extrapyramidal syndromes.

Baldessarini (1990) has enumerated six types of extrapyramidal syndromes associated with the use of antipsychotic drugs.

Effects Usually Appearing during Drug Administration

Acute Dystonic Reactions

The period of maximum risk is within hours to 5 days after initiation of neuroleptic therapy. There may also be increased risk following increments in dose. High-potency, low-dose antipsychotics are more likely to precipitate an acute dystonic reaction than are low-potency, high-dose antipsychotics, and young males, both children and adolescents, may be at increased risk (APA, 1980b). Untreated acute dystonic reactions may last from a few minutes to several hours, and they may recur. Symptoms, which may be painful and frightening, particularly if the patient does not understand what is happening, include muscular hypertonicity; tonic contractions (spasms) of the neck (torticollis), mouth, and tongue (which may make speaking difficult); oculogyric crisis (eyes rolling upward and remaining in that position); and opisthotonos (spasm in which the spine and extremities are bend with a forward convexity). Acute dystonic reactions respond rapidly to anticholinergic and antiparkinsonian drugs, such as diphenhydramine (Benadryl) 25 to 50 mg orally or intramuscularly or benztropine (Cogentin) 1 to 2 mg intramuscularly. (The manufacturer of benztropine cautions that its use is contraindicated in children under 3 years of age and that it should be used with caution in older children [PDR, 1990]). If the dystonia is very severe, administering either 25 mg of diphenhydramine intramuscularly or 1 to 2 mg of benztropine intramuscularly will reverse the dystonia within a few minutes. The prophylactic use of anticholinergic and antiparkinsonian agents to prevent acute dystonic reactions is discussed below, following the section on akathisia.

Parkinsonism (Pseudoparkinsonism)

The period of maximum risk is 5 to 30 days after initiation of neuroleptic therapy. The risk for development of parkinsonism appears to be greater for females and to increase with age. It is rarely seen in preschool children treated with therapeutic doses of neuroleptics; it occurs commonly in school-age children and adolescents (Campbell et al., 1985). Symptoms include tremor, cogwheel rigidity, drooling, and decrease in facial expressive movements (mask-like or expressionless facies) and akinesia (slowness in initiating movements). These symptoms respond to antiparkinsonian medication; for example, benztropine (Cogentin) 1 to 2 mg given two or three times daily usually provides relief within a day or two. Antiparkinsonian medication may be withdrawn after a week or two to see if it is still necessary for symptomatic relief.

Akinesia, perhaps the most severe form of parkinsonism, is defined by Rifkin et al. (1975) as a "behavioral state of diminished spontaneity characterized by few gestures, unspontaneous speech and, particularly, apathy and difficulty with initiating usual activities" (p. 672). It may be particularly difficult to differentiate from the negative symptoms of schizophrenia, such as apathy and blunting. Van Putten et al. (1987) considered that akinesia might be the most toxic behavioral side effect of antipsychotic drugs. The authors noted that a subjective sense of sedation or drowsiness, excessive sleeping, and a lack of any leg-crossing during an interview of about 20 minutes correlated with the presence of akinesia. Akinesia also interferes with social adjustment, and the patient may appear to have a "postpsychotic depression." Patients with akinesia often are less concerned with any psychotic symptoms and report that everything is all right; they may experience an absence of emotion and appear emotionally dead (Van Putten et al., 1987). Although antiparkinsonian drugs may be helpful, in some cases they do not adequately control symptoms of akinesia. There is some evidence that antiparkinsonian drugs become less effective at higher daily dosages of antipsychotics (Van Putten et al., 1987).

The prophylactic use of anticholinergic and antiparkinsonian agents to prevent pseudoparkinsonism is discussed below, following the section on akathisia.

Akathisia (Motor Restlessness)

The period of maximum risk for developing this condition is 5 to 60 days after initiation of neuroleptic therapy, but it has been reported to occur in as few as 6 hours after an oral dose of a neuroleptic (Van Putten et al., 1984). Symptoms include constant uncomfortable restlessness, a feeling of tension in the lower extremities often accompanied by a strong or irresistible urge to move them, inability to sit still, and foot-tapping or pacing. Clinically, blunted affect, emotional withdrawal, and motor retardation may also be observed (Van Putten et al., 1987).

Akathisia may or may not respond to antiparkinsonian drugs

such as trihexyphenidyl (Artane). Van Putten et al. (1987) noted the dual nature of akathisia: a subjective experience of restlessness and observable motor restlessness. In their clinical experience, all patients with moderate or severe akathisia exhibited either rocking from foot to foot or walking on the spot. Akathisia was also strongly associated with depression, dysphoria, and, at times in severe and treatment-resistant cases, with exacerbation of psychotic symptoms and homicidal and suicidal ideation and behavior (Van Putten et al., 1987). Of particular clinical importance, patients who have unpleasant untoward effects, especially akathisia, with antipsychotics are more likely to be noncompliant and to unilaterally discontinue medication early in treatment (Van Putten et al., 1987).

Fleischhacker et al. (1989) have published a rating scale for akathisia that includes two subjective items: "a sensation of inner restlessness" and "the urge to move" and three items that characterize the frequency and magnitude of observed akathisia phenomena.

Propranolol may be helpful in ameliorating akathisia (Adler et al., 1986); benzodiazepines and clonidine have also been reported to be effective in some cases.

Clonazepam was administered to 10 first-onset psychotic adolescents (8 of whom were diagnosed with schizophrenia, paranoid subtype) between 16 and 19 years of age who experienced distressing akathisia following treatment with antipsychotics (Kutcher et al., 1987). Nine of the patients also had been receiving benztropine concomitantly with their antipsychotic medication. All patients reported subjective improvement, and scores on an akathisia subscale decreased significantly after a week's treatment with 0.5 mg/day of clonazepam.

In some cases, reduction in dose of the antipsychotic may be necessary. Neppe and Ward (1989) recommend that if only akathisia develops (i.e., without accompanying parkinsonism) that a β-blocker be used rather than an anticholinergic agent.

The Prophylactic Use of Antiparkinsonian Agents for Acute Dystonic Reaction, Parkinsonism, and Akathisia

The use of antiparkinsonian (anticholinergic) agents prophylactically to minimize the likelihood of the patient's developing an acute dystonic reaction, parkinsonism, or akathisia from antipsychotics is controversial. Some of the reasons for this have to do with the effects caused by the anticholinergic agents themselves. Anticholinergic agents may affect cognition adversely and may aggravate psychotic symptomatology. In addition, there is some suggestion that at least part of the effectiveness of these agents is that they may lower the serum concentration of the antipsychotic (Rivera-Calimlim et al., 1976). Because of their reluctance to give an additional medication that itself may have untoward effects, many clinicians choose to minimize the risk of these extrapyramidal effects by beginning with a low dose and titrating the medication slowly. If an acute dystonic reaction should occur, it may be treated with diphenhydramine and the dosage of antipsychotic lowered temporarily if necessary. On the other hand, some clinicians routinely prescribe an agent such as benztropine for approximately a month to 6 weeks, covering the period of maximal risk for the development of both acute dystonic reactions and parkinsonian untoward effects. Another option for outpatients is to prescribe a small amount of an anticholinergic (e.g., diphenhydramine), with an explanation of how it is to be administered should such a reaction occur (e.g., to take one capsule should a dystonic reaction begin, to take another dose in 20 to 30 minutes if there is no improvement, and to go to an emergency room if the reaction is severe and alert the physician to the medication being taken).

In their recent review of the management of acute extrapyramidal syndromes induced by neuroleptics, Neppe and Ward (1989) note that anticholinergics can significantly reduce the rate of acute dystonias, especially in the highest-risk group, males under 30 years of age treated with high-potency antipsychotics. However, as acute dystonic reactions tend to be transient, prophylactic treatment for more than 2 weeks is not usually indicated. These authors recommend no prophylaxis for parkinsonism and akathisia, as they rarely present as dramatically emergent a picture as acute dystonia. The parents and/or patient as appropriate may be carefully informed about the possibility of these conditions arising, to aid in their early detection. The clinician can then decide how best to treat the particular symptom in the particular patient (Neppe & Ward, 1989).

Van Putten et al. (1987) point out that prophylactic use of antiparkinsonian drugs may not fully prevent symptoms of akinesia from developing and that some schizophrenic patients who have been stabilized using antiparkinsonian medication may experience increased anxiety, depression, general dysphoria and suffering when the anticholinergics are withdrawn.

The clinician should decide on a case-by-case basis which of the above possibilities is best for a given patient. This will be based on factors such as whether a high- or low-potency neuroleptic is given, how rapidly the dose is to be increased, previous experience of the patient, whether it is administered to an outpatient or to an inpatient where clinical staff are readily available, how such a reaction might affect the relationship with patient and/or parents and subsequent compliance, and the patient's environment. For example, it can be particularly difficult for a patient and family if the patient develops an acute dystonic reaction while attending school.

Neuroleptic Malignant Syndrome

This condition is life threatening and can occur within weeks after initiation of neuroleptic therapy; males and younger adults appear to be most often affected (for review see Kaufmann & Wyatt, 1987). Symptoms include severe muscular rigidity, altered consciousness, stupor, catatonia, hyperpyrexia, labile pulse and blood pressure, and occasionally myoglobinemia. It can persist for up to 2 weeks or longer after medication is discontinued and can be fatal. Treatment consists of immediate cessation of medication and hospitalization with supportive treatment. Antiparkinsonian drugs are not useful.

Late-Appearing Syndromes (after Months or Years of Treatment)

Tardive Dyskinesia

Definitions and descriptions of tardive dyskinesia and related dyskinesias (withdrawal, masked dyskinesias) vary. Perhaps the most influential definition at the present time is the research diagnostic criteria proposed in 1982 by Schooler and Kane. They note that if possible, the absence of abnormal involuntary movements prior to beginning pharmacotherapy should be documented. Schooler and Kane (1982) proposed three prerequisites for making the diagnosis, which are summarized as follows:

1. exposure to neuroleptics for a minimum total cumulative exposure of 3 months
2. the presence of at least "moderate" abnormal involuntary movements in one or more body areas (face, lips, jaw, tongue, upper extremities, lower extremities, trunk) and at least "mild" movements in two or more body areas

3. absence of other conditions that might produce abnormal movements

Tardive dyskinesia develops while actively receiving a neuroleptic, as opposed to a withdrawal dyskinesia that occurs when a neuroleptic is withdrawn or its dose is decreased. Tardive dyskinesia, which may be both severely disabling and irreversible, is the most clinically significant common long-term untoward effect of antipsychotics. Baldessarini (1990) notes that in some cases, especially in younger patients, tardive dyskinesia will disappear over the course of weeks to as much as 3 years. It is believed that the risk of developing irreversible tardive dyskinesia increases with both total cumulative dose and duration of treatment. Older females appear to be at increased risk. It has been reported that fine worm-like (vermicular) movements of the tongue may be an early sign of tardive dyskinesia, and that discontinuation of the medication when this occurs may prevent further development of the syndrome (PDR, 1990). Symptoms of tardive dyskinesia most typically include involuntary choreoathetotic movements affecting the face; tongue; perioral, buccal, and masticatory musculature; and neck, but which may also involve the torso and extremities.

Atypical and less common forms of tardive dyskinesia, such as tardive akathisia, a persisting restlessness, and tardive dystonia, also occur. Burke et al. (1982) reported 42 cases of tardive dystonia that they diagnosed by the following criteria:

1. the presence of chronic dystonia
2. history of antipsychotic drug treatment preceding or concurrent with the onset of dystonia
3. exclusion of known causes of secondary dystonia by appropriate clincial and laboratory evaluation
4. a negative family history for dystonia

Symptoms of tardive dystonia began after as few as 3 days and up to 11 years after initiation of antipsychotic medication. The incidence of tardive dystonia was more frequent in younger male patients than in older patients; was characterized by sustained abnormal postures accompanied by torticollis, torsion of the trunk and extremities, blepharospasm, and grimacing; and was incapacitating in severe cases. Spontaneous remission occurred in a few patients, but in most dystonia persisted for years. Of the many medications used in an attempt to ameliorate the tardive dystonia, the most helpful were tetrabenzine, which improved symptoms in

68% of patients, and anticholinergics, which were helpful in 39% of patients (Burke et al., 1982). In tardive dyskinesia and other choreoathetotic syndromes, typically emotional stress causes worsening of the movements, drowsiness or sedation causes them to diminish, and they disappear during sleep (APA, 1980b). There is no adequate treatment; antiparkinsonian drugs may worsen the condition (for review see APA, 1980b).

In addition, a withdrawal dyskinesia may emerge when neuroleptic medication is withdrawn or the dose is reduced. Withdrawal-emergent dyskinesias can occur for two different reasons: First, antidopaminergic drugs, including antipsychotics, can suppress tardive dyskinesia; thus decreasing their serum levels can "unmask" ongoing tardive dyskinesia. Second, Baldessarini (1990) points out that a "disuse supersensitivity" to dopamine agonists may also occur following withdrawal of antidopaminergic drugs and suggests that this phenomenon may explain withdrawal dyskinesias that resolve within a few weeks.

The reported prevalence of neuroleptic-induced tardive and withdrawal dyskinesias in children has ranged from 8% to 51% (for review see Campbell et al., 1983). If tardive dyskinesia develops, every effort should be made to discontinue or at least reduce the dose of antipsychotic as much as possible. The dyskinesia should be monitored with serial ratings on the AIMS. Experience suggests that a large percentage of tardive and withdrawal dyskinesias that develop in children are reversible if the drug is stopped. If the severity of the psychiatric disorder precludes discontinuation of antipsychotic medication (e.g., in a patient with autistic disorder with severe self-injurious behavior and aggressiveness who has not responded adequately to other medications such as lithium or propranolol), the clinician must carefully document the rationale for reinstituting antipsychotic medication and that the legal guardians (and patient when appropriate) have given their informed consent. Reinstating or increasing the dose of antipsychotic may suppress or mask tardive dyskinesia.

Because of such risks, antipsychotics should be given only to children and adolescents for whom no other potentially less harmful treatment is available; for example, while effective in some children diagnosed with ADHD, antipsychotics should not be used unless stimulant medications, and probably imipramine and desipramine too, have been treatment failures.

Although antipsychotics are the only drugs that result in persistent tardive dyskinesia in a significant proportion of patients, a number of different drugs may cause dyskinesias after short- or long-term treatment. Jeste and Wyatt (1982) note that the dyskinesia produced by L-dopa most closely resembles the tardive dyskinesia resulting from antipsychotics and that, typically, the dyskinesias caused by most other drugs are usually acute, sometimes toxic, effects and almost always remit when the drug is discontinued. Among the drugs used in child and adolescent psychopharmacotherapy for which dyskinesias have been reported are amphetamines, methylphenidate, monoamine oxidase inhibitors, tricyclic antidepressants, lithium, antihistamines, benzodiazepines, and antiepileptic drugs (Jeste & Wyatt, 1982).

Rabbit Syndrome (Perioral Tremor)

This condition, which may be a late-onset variant of parkinsonism, is uncommon. Its name derives from the fact that patients so afflicted make rapid chewing movements similar to those of rabbits (Villeneuve, 1972). It may respond to antiparkinsonian medication.

Other Untoward Effects of Antipsychotics

Table 4.1 is a compilation of most of the reported untoward effects of chlorpromazine, the prototype drug of the antipsychotics. Most of these untoward effects have also been reported to occur to a greater or lesser degree with other antipsychotics.

REPRESENTATIVE ANTIPSYCHOTICS USED IN CHILD AND ADOLESCENT PSYCHIATRY

Table 4.2 summarizes representative antipsychotic drugs commonly used in child and adolescent psychiatry. It compares their relative potencies and expectable potential sedative, autonomic, and extrapyramidal untoward effects with chlorpromazine, the prototype of the antipsychotics. FDA age limitations and recommended dosages for approved use in children and adolescents are also given when available.

Although it is usually recommended that antipsychotics initially be administered in divided doses, most frequently three or four times daily, once the optimal dose is established, their relatively long serum half-lives usually permit either once daily dosage (e.g., before bedtime) or twice daily dosage, in the morning and before bedtime.

Table 4.1.
Untoward Effects of Chlorpromazine

Allergic
   Mild urticaria
   Photosensitivity, exfoliative dermatitis
   Asthma
   Anaphylactoid reactions
   Laryngeal edema
   Angioneurotic Edema
Autonomic nervous system
   Antiadrenergic effects
      Orthostatic hypotension
      Ejaculatory disturbances
   Anticholinergic effects
      Decreased secretion, resulting in dry mouth, dry eyes, nasal congestion
      Blurred vision, mydriasis
      Glaucoma attack in patients with narrow-angle closure
      Constipation, paralytic ileus
      Urinary retention
      Impotence
Cardiovascular
   Postural (orthostatic) hypotension
   Tachycardia
   ECG changes
   Sudden death due to cardiac arrest
Central nervous system
   Neuromuscular effects
      Dystonias
      Akasthisia (motor restlessness)
      Pseudoparkinsonism
      Tardive dyskinesia
   Seizures, lowering of seizure threshold
   Drowsiness, sedation
   Behavioral effects
      Increased psychotic symptoms
      Catatonic-like states
Dermatological
   Photosensitivity
   Skin pigmentation changes in exposed areas
   Rashes
Endocrinological
   Elevated prolactin levels
   Gynecomastia
   Amenorrhea
   Hyperglycemia, glycosuria, and hypoglycemia
Hematological
   Agranulocytosis
   Eosinophilia
   Leukopenia

(continued)

Table 4.1. continued
Untoward Effects of Chlorpromazine

Hemolytic anemia
Aplastic anemia
Thrombocytopenic purpura
Pancytopenia
Hepatological
  Jaundice
Metabolic
  Weight gain, increased appetite
Ophthalmologic
  Blurred vision
  Precipitation of acute glaucoma attack in persons with narrow-angle glaucoma
  Deposition of pigmented material and star-shaped opacities in lens
  Deposition of pigmented material in cornea
  Pigmentary retinopathy
  Epithelial keratopathy
Teratogenic effects possible (seen in animal studies)
Other
  Neuroleptic malignant syndrome
  Sudden death, which may be related to cardiac failure or suppression of
    cough reflex

Chlorpromazine (Thorazine)

Indications in Child and Adolescent Psychiatry
    In addition to being approved for uses similar to those for adults, including psychotic disorders, it is approved for the treatment of severe behavioral problems in children, marked by combativeness and/or explosive hyperexcitable behavior. It is also noted that dosages over 500 mg/day are unlikely to further enhance behavioral improvement in severely disturbed mentally retarded patients.
    Chlorpromazine may lower the threshold to seizures; another antipsychotic should be chosen for seizure-prone individuals.
- Infants under 6 months of age: Not recommended.
- Children over 6 months to 12 years of age with severe behavioral problems or psychotic conditions:
  Oral: 0.25 mg/kg every 4 to 6 hours as needed. Titrate upward gradually. In severe cases daily doses of 200 mg or higher may be required.
  Rectal: 1 mg/kg every 6 to 8 hours as needed.
  Intramuscular: 0.5 mg/kg every 6 to 8 hours as needed. Maximum daily intramuscular dose for a child under 5 years or under 22 kg is 40 mg; for a child 5 to 12 years of age or 22 kg to 45 kg, maximum daily dose is 75 mg.

- Adolescents: Depending on severity of symptoms, begin with 10 mg three times to 25 mg four times daily. Titrate upward with increases of 20 to 50 mg twice weekly. For severely agitated patients, 25 mg intramuscularly may be given and repeated if necessary in 1 hour. Any subsequent intramuscular medication should be at 4- to 6-hour intervals.

Dose Forms Available
- Tablets: 10 mg, 25 mg, 50 mg, 100 mg, 200 mg
- Syrup: 10 mg/5 ml
- Suppositories 25 mg, 100 mg
- Concentrate: 30 mg/ml, 100 mg/ml
- Injectable: 25 mg/ml

Thioridazine (Mellaril)

Indications in Child and Adolescent Psychiatry

In addition to psychotic disorders, thioridazine has FDA approval for treating severe behavioral problems marked by combativeness and/or explosive hyperexcitable behavior (out of proportion to immediate provocations), and in the short-term treatment of hyperactive children who show excessive motor activity with accompanying conduct disorders consisting of some or all of the following symptoms: impulsivity, difficulty sustaining attention, aggressivity, mood lability, and poor frustration tolerance.

Dosage Schedule for Children and Adolescents
- Children under 2 years of age: Not recommended.
- Children 2 to 12 years of age: Usual dosage ranges from 0.5 mg/kg/day to a maximum of 3 mg/kg/day. Start with a low dose and titrate upward for optimal therapeutic effect. More severely disturbed children may initially require 25 mg two or three times daily.
- Older adolescents: As in adults, a maximum of 800 mg/day is permitted to minimize the likelihood that pigmentary retinopathy will develop. The initial dose depends on the severity of the disorder; frequently 25 mg to 50 mg two or three times daily is an appropriate starting dosage.

Dose Forms Available
- Tablets: 10 mg, 15 mg, 25 mg, 50 mg, 100 mg, 150 mg, 200 mg
- Concentrate: 30 mg/ml, 100 mg/ml
- Suspension: 25 mg/5 ml, 100 mg/5 ml

Table 4.2.
Antipsychotic Drugs[a]

Drug	Chemical Classification	Therapeutically Equivalent Oral Dose (mg)	Effects			Approved Age for Use	Usual Optimal Dose/ Maintenance Dose Range
			Sedation	Autonomic[b]	Extrapyramidal Reaction[c]		
Chlorpromazine[d] Thorazine (Smith Kline & French)	Phenothiazine: aliphatic compound	100	+++	+++	++	Over 6 months	See text
Chlorprothixene Taractan (Roche)	Thioxanthene	100	+++	+++	+/++	Over 6 years	10 to 25 mg 3 to 4 times daily
Thioridazine[d] Mellaril (Sandoz)	Phenothiazine: piperidine compound	100	+++	+++	+	2 years	See text
Clozapine Clozaril (Sandoz)	Dibenzodiazepine	75	+++	+++	0?	16 years	As per adults See text
Mesoridazine Serentil (Boehringer Ingelheim)	Phenothiazine: piperidine compound	50	+++	++	+	12 years	No specific doses for children
Loxapine[d] Loxitane (Lederle)	Dibenzoxazepine	15	++	+/++	++/+++	16 years	As per adults

Molindone Moban (DuPont)	Dihydroindolone	10	++	+	+	12 years	No specific doses for children
Perphenazine[d] Trilafon (Schering)	Phenothiazine: piperazine compound	10	++	+	++/+++	12 years	No specific doses for children
Trifluoperazine[d] Stelazine (Smith Kline & French)	Phenothiazine: piperazine compound	5	++	+	+++	6 years	See text
Thiothixene[d] Navane (Roerig)	Thioxanthene	5	+	+	+++	12 years	No specific doses for children
Fluphenazine[d] Permitil (Schering) Prolixin (Princeton)	Phenothiazine: piperazine compound	2	+	+	+++	16 years	See text
Haloperidol[d] Haldol (McNeil)	Butyrophenone	2	+	+	+++	3 years	See text
Pimozide[e] Orap (Lemmon)	Diphenylbutyl-piperidine	10	+	+	+++	Over 12 years	0.2 mg/kg/day or maximum, 10 mg/day

[a] Adapted from American Medical Association. Drug Evaluations. Chicago: American Medical Association, 1990.

[b] Alpha antiadrenergic and anticholinergic effects.

[c] Excluding tardive dyskinesia, which appears to be produced to the same degree and frequency by all agents with equieffective antipsychotic doses (except clozapine).

[d] Available generically.

[e] Only indicated for Tourette's disorder that has not responded to other standard treatments; not approved for use in psychoses.

Trifluoperazine (Stelazine)

Indications in Child and Adolescent Psychiatry
One manufacturer has a specific disclaimer that trifluoperazine has not been proven effective in the management of behavioral complications in patients with mental retardation and recommends it only for the treatment of psychotic individuals and the short-term treatment of nonpsychotic anxiety in individuals with generalized anxiety disorder who have not responded to other medications.

Dosage Schedule for Children and Adolescents
- Children under 6 years of age: Not recommended.
- Children 6 to 12 years of age: A starting dose of 1 mg once or twice daily with gradual upward titration is recommended. Dosages in excess of 15 mg/day are usually required only by older children with severe symptoms.
- Adolescents: 1 to 5 mg twice daily. Usually the optimal dose will be 15 to 20 mg/day at most; occasionally up to 40 mg/day will be required. Titration to optimal dose can usually be accomplished within 2 to 3 weeks.

Dose Forms Available
- Tablets: 1 mg, 2 mg, 5 mg, 10 mg
- Concentrate: 10 mg/ml
- Injectable: 2 mg/ml (One manufacturer notes there is little experience using intramuscular trifluoperazine with children and recommends 1 mg intramuscularly once, or maximally twice, daily if necessary for rapid control of severe symptoms.)

Haloperidol (Haldol)

Indications in Child and Adolescent Psychiatry
Haloperidol is approved for the treatment of psychotic disorders and Tourette's disorder. Only after the failure of treatment with psychotherapy and non-antipsychotic medications has haloperidol been approved for treating children with severe behavioral disorders—for example, "combative, explosive hyperexcitability (which cannot be accounted for by immediate provocation)" (package insert)—and the short-term treatment of hyperactive children with coexisting conduct disorders who exhibit such symptoms as "impulsivity, difficulty sustaining attention, aggressivity, mood liability and poor frustration tolerance)" (package insert).
Shapiro and Shapiro (1989) concluded that the most effective neuroleptics in the treatment of tics and Tourette's disorder were halo-

peridol, pimozide (Orap), fluphenazine (Prolixin, Permitil), and penfluridol (Semap, an investigational drug).

Dosage Schedule for Children and Adolescents with Psychotic Disorders, Tourette's Disorder, or Severe Nonpsychotic Behavioral Disorders

- Children under 3 years of age: Not recommended.
- Children 3 to 12 years of age (weight, 15 to 40 kg): Begin with 0.5 mg daily; titrate upward by 0.5 mg increments at 5- to 7-day intervals.
- Therapeutic dose ranges are usually from 0.05 to 0.075 mg/kg/day for nonpsychotic behavioral disorders and Tourette's disorder; for psychotic children the upper range is usually 0.15 mg/kg/day but may be higher in severe cases. Morselli et al. (1983) reported good therapeutic results in children with tics and Tourette's disorder associated with haloperidol plasma levels in the range of 1 to 3 ng/ml. Higher haloperidol plasma levels, usually between 6 and 10 ng/ml, were necessary for significant improvement in psychotic conditions.
- Adolescents (over age 12): Depending on severity 0.5 to 5 mg two or three times daily. Higher doses may be necessary for more rapid control in some severe cases.

Dose Forms Available

- Tablets: 0.5 mg, 1 mg, 2 mg, 5 mg, 10 mg, 20 mg
- Concentrate solution: 2 mg/ml
- Injectable (haloperidol decanoate): Safety not established for children. If necessary, in acutely agitated adolescents an initial dose of 2 to 5 mg may be given intramuscularly. Additional medication may be given every 1 to 8 hours as determined by ongoing evaluation of the patient.

Pharmacokinetics of Haloperidol

Morselli et al. (1983) noted that steady-state haloperidol plasma levels in children may vary up to 15-fold at a given mg/kg daily dosage, but for a given individual the relationship between dosage and plasma level is fairly consistent. Most children had haloperidol plasma half-lives that were shorter than those of adolescents and adults. The authors also emphasized, however, that despite their more rapid metabolism of haloperidol, children did not require proportionally higher daily doses as they also appear to be more sensitive to both the therapeutic and the untoward effects of haloperidol at lower plasma concentrations than were older adolescents and adults (Morselli et al., 1983).

Haloperidol in the Treatment of Autistic Disorder

At the present time, haloperidol is the most well-studied drug used in the treatment of autistic disorder and is recommended as the drug of first choice. In a study of 40 autistic children aged 2.33 to 6.92 years, haloperidol in optimal doses of 0.5 to 3 mg/day yielded global clinical improvement and decreased significantly symptoms of withdrawal, stereotypies, abnormal object relationships, hyperactivity, fidgetiness, negativism, and angry and labile affect (Anderson et al., 1984). A high rate of dyskinesias, however, remains a problem. Significant numbers of autistic children (22%, or 8 of 36) developed tardive dyskinesia or withdrawal dyskinesia in a prospective study in which 0.5 to 3 mg/day of haloperidol were administered for from $3^{1}/_{2}$ to $42^{1}/_{2}$ months, so close monitoring is necessary (Perry et al., 1985).

In autistic disorder, stereotypies existing at baseline may be suppressed by administration of haloperidol. When the drug is withdrawn, there is potential for confusion between the reappearance of stereotypies and a withdrawal dyskinesia; this is of special concern if a physician unfamiliar with the child at baseline assumes treatment responsibilities for the child while he or she is on maintenance medication.

Haloperidol in the Treatment of Childhood-Onset and Atypical Pervasive Developmental Disorders

Joshi et al. (1988) administered fluphenazine or haloperidol to 12 children aged 7 to 11 years who were hospitalized and diagnosed with childhood-onset or atypical pervasive developmental disorders (PDDs) (i.e., approximately equivalent to the DSM-III-R [1987] diagnoses of autistic disorder with childhood onset and PDD not otherwise specified [PDDNOS]). The children responded with remarkable improvement in peer interactions and reality testing and decreases in autistic-like behavior, aggressiveness, impulsivity, and hyperactivity. Seven of the 12 children were able to return home rather than be admitted to residential treatment as had been planned. Haloperidol was begun at a dose of 0.02 mg/kg/day and titrated based on behavioral response, with increases at 3- to 5-day intervals. Mean optimal dose of haloperidol was 0.04 ± 0.01 mg/kg/day. Untoward effects were remarkably infrequent. Drowsiness occurred initially in some children but it was transient and did not interfere with their later cognitive performance. Two children receiving haloperidol developed some rigidity and cogwheeling that responded to oral diphenhydramine during the first few days of treatment; the extra-pyramidal symptoms did not recur when the diphenhydramine was discontinued.

Haloperidol in the Treatment of Aggressive Conduct Disorder

In a double-blind placebo-controlled study of 61 treatment-resistant hospitalized children aged 5.2 to 12.9 years with under-socialized aggressive conduct disorder, both haloperidol and lithium were found to be superior to placebo in ameliorating behavioral symptoms (Campbell et al., 1984b). Optimal doses of haloperidol ranged from 1 to 6 mg/day. The authors reported that at optimal doses, the untoward effects of haloperidol appeared to interfere more significantly with the children's daily routines than did those of lithium.

Thiothixene (Navane)

Indications in Child and Adolescent Psychiatry

Thiothixene is an antipsychotic drug of the thioxanthene series. It is indicated in the management of symptoms of psychotic disorders. It has not been evaluated in the management of behavioral disturbances in the mentally retarded, nor is its use recommended in children under age 12 years as safe conditions for its use in that age group have not been established (PDR, 1990).

Dosage Schedule for Children and Adolescents at Least 12 Years Old

• Milder conditions: Initial dose of 2 mg three times daily with titration to 5 mg three times daily if needed is usually effective.
• More severe conditions: Initial dose of 5 mg twice daily. The usual optimal dose is 20 to 30 mg/day; occasionally up to 60 mg/day are required. Daily doses of over 60 mg rarely increase the beneficial response (PDR, 1990).

Dose Forms Available

• Capsules: 1 mg, 2 mg, 5 mg, 10 mg, 20 mg
• Concentrate: 5 mg/ml
• Intramuscular: 2 mg/ml

Investigational Report of Interest

Realmuto and his colleagues (1984) assigned 21 adolescent (mean age, 15.1 years; range, 11.75 to 18.33 years) chronic schizo-phrenic inpatients to either thiothixene or thioridazine. Optimal dose was individually titrated over a period of about 2 weeks. For the 13 patients who received thiothixene, the mean optimal dose was 16.2 mg/day (range, 4.8 to 42.6 mg/day) or 0.30 mg/kg/day for 4 to 6 weeks. Hallucinations, anxiety, tension, and excitement decreased the most during the 1st week. Cognitive disorganization improved more slowly. There were no significant differences between the two drugs and rapidity of symptom improvement or extent of improvement at the end of the study. About 50% of patients improved, regardless of the medication. There was a suggestion, however, that untoward effects, particularly drowsiness, were less severe with thiothixene than with thioridazine and that because of this, high-potency antipsychotics may be preferable to the more sedating low-potency antipsychotics in treating adolescent schizophrenics (Realmuto et al., 1984).

Chlorprothixene (Taractan)

Indications in Child and Adolescent Psychiatry
   Chlorprothixene is a thioxanthene antipsychotic that has been approved by the FDA for oral administration to persons over 6 years of age in the management of psychotic disorders. Parenteral use is not approved for persons under 12 years of age. The manufacturer notes that chlorprothixene has not been proven efficacious in treating behavioral disturbances in the mentally retarded.

Dosage Schedule for Treating Psychotic Disorders in Children and Adolescents
• Children under 6 years of age: Not approved.
• Children over 6 years of age and younger adolescents: 10 to 25 mg three or four times daily.

Dose Forms Available
• Tablets: 10 mg, 25 mg, 50 mg, 100 mg
• Concentrate: 100 mg/5 ml
• Intramuscular: 25 mg/2 ml

Loxapine Succinate (Loxitane)

Indications in Child and Adolescent Psychiatry
   Loxapine is a dibenzoxazepine compound with antipsychotic properties used in treating psychotic disorders. The manufacturer does not recommend its use in persons under 16 years of age.

Dosage Schedule for Children and Adolescents
- Children and adolescents under 16 years old: Not recommended.
- Adolescents at least 16 years old and adults: An initial dose of 10 mg twice daily is recommended and is titrated according to clinical response. The usual therapeutic and maintenance dose ranges from 60 to 100 mg daily. A maximum of 250 mg/day is recommended.

Dose Forms Available
- Capsules: 5 mg, 10 mg, 25 mg, 50 mg
- Oral concentrate: 25 mg/ml
- Injection (Intramuscular): 50 mg/ml

Investigational Report of Interest

Pool and colleagues (1976) conducted a 4-week double-blind study comparing the efficacies of loxapine, haloperidol, and placebo in 75 adolescents 13 to 18 years of age diagnosed with acute schizophrenia or chronic schizophrenia with an acute exacerbation. Loxapine was begun at a dose of 10 mg daily and titrated to a maximum of 200 mg daily (average daily dose, 87.5 mg). Extrapyramidal reactions, most commonly parkinsonian muscular rigidity, were the most frequent untoward effects of loxapine and occurred in 19 of 26 subjects. The second most frequent untoward effect, sedation, occurred in 21 of the 26 subjects. Both loxapine and haloperidol were significantly superior to placebo in diminishing schizophrenic symptoms. The authors concluded that loxapine was relatively safe and efficacious in the treatment of adolescent schizophrenia.

Fluphenazine Hydrochloride (Prolixin, Permitil)

Indications in Child and Adolescent Psychiatry
Fluphenazine hydrochloride is approved for the treatment of psychotic disorders. It is, however, not approved for administration to children under age 12 years because of a lack of studies proving its efficacy and safety in this age group. A manufacturer notes that it has not been shown to be effective in treating behaviorally disturbed patients who are mentally retarded.

Dose Schedule for Children and Adolescents
- Children under 12 years of age: Not recommended.
- Children at least 12 years of age and adolescents: Manufacturer recommends an initial total daily dose of 2.5 to 10 mg divided and administered every 6 to 8 hours for adults. One should be at least this conservative in adolescents (see also Joshi et al. [1988] below).

Dose Forms Available
- Tablets: 1 mg, 2.5 mg, 5 mg, 10 mg
- Elixir: 0.5 mg/ml (2.5 mg/5 ml)
- Injectable: (Fluphenazine hydrochloride): 2.5 mg/ml
- Oral concentrate: 5 mg/ml
- Long-acting preparations for parenteral administration: fluphenazine enanthate, 25 mg/ml, and fluphenazine decanoate, 25 mg/ml, are available. (They are used primarily in treating adults diagnosed with chronic schizophrenia.)

Investigational Report of Interest

As discussed above under "Haloperidol," Joshi et al. (1988) found fluphenazine to be efficacious in treating children diagnosed with childhood-onset PDD or atypical PDD. Fluphenazine was begun at 0.02 mg/kg/day and increased at 3- to 5-day intervals, based on behavioral responses. Mean optimal dose of fluphenazine was 1.3 ± 0.7 mg/day. Untoward effects of fluphenazine were remarkably infrequent. Some initial drowsiness occurred but it was transient.

Pimozide (Orap)

Indications in Child and Adolescent Psychiatry
Pimozide is an antipsychotic drug of the diphenylbutylpiperidine series. It is indicated only in the treatment of patients with Tourette's disorder whose development and/or daily life function is severely compromised by the presence of motor and phonic tics and who have not responded satisfactorily to or cannot tolerate standard treatments, such as haloperidol. There is limited experience with its use in children under 12 years of age.

Dosage Schedule for Children and Adolescents
As there is very limited information available on the use of pimozide in children, it should be introduced at a very low dose and gradually adjusted upward. It is suggested that treatment should be initiated with 0.5 mg/day and gradually increased by increments of 0.5 mg once or twice weekly.

Most patients are maintained at less than 0.2 mg/kg/day or 10 mg/day, whichever is less. Doses greater than 0.2 mg/kg/day or 10 mg/day are not recommended. Unexplained deaths, perhaps cardiac related, and grand mal seizures have occurred in patients taking high doses of pimozide (over 20 mg/day) (PDR, 1990).

Dose Forms Available
- Scored tablets: 2 mg

Pharmacokinetics of Pimozide

Peak serum levels usually occur 6 to 8 hours after ingestion of pimozide. Pimozide is metabolized primarily in the liver; it and its metabolites are excreted primarily through the kidneys. There are wide interindividual variations in half-life and in peak serum levels for equivalent doses. Mean serum half-life in schizophrenics was about 55 hours. There are few correlations between plasma levels and clinical findings (package insert).

Untoward Effects of Pimozide

Pimozide prolongs the Q-T interval of the ECG. An ECG should be done at baseline and monthly during the period of dose titration. Increase of the Q-T interval beyond an absolute limit of 0.47 second in children or 0.52 second in adults or more than 25% above the patient's original baseline should be considered a mandate for no further increase in dose and for possibly lowering the dose. Because hypokalemia is associated with ventricular arrhythmias, potassium levels should be monitored during therapy.

Contraindications for Pimozide Administration

In addition to considerations for antipsychotics in general, pimozide is contraindicated in the treatment of simple tics or tics other than those associated with Tourette's disorder. Pimozide also should not be given to patients with congenital long Q-T intervals or a history of cardiac arrhythmias.

Use of Pimozide in Children and Adolescents with Treatment-Resistant Tourette's Disorder

Shapiro, Shapiro, and Eisenkraft (1983) treated 31 patients aged 10 to 50 years (mean age, 19.6 ± 9.2 years) diagnosed with Tourette's syndrome with pimozide in an open study. All had previously received haloperidol and either had unsatisfactory symptom control, an unacceptable level of untoward effects, or a desire to try pimozide. Pimozide was titrated in 1-mg increments every 4 to 7 days until optimal dose was achieved. The mean optimal dose of pimozide was 12.9 ± 12.5 mg/day (median dose, 8 mg/day; range, 1 to 64 mg/day). In this subgroup of patients, the therapeutic efficacy of pimozide was superior to that of haloperidol. Significantly more patients treated with pimozide (74.4%) achieved more than 70% symptomatic improvement than with haloperidol (45.4%). The mean score for untoward effects was significantly less for pimozide than for haloperidol. The authors hypothesized that the superiority of pimozide was related to its relative lack of norepinephrine antagonism compared to halo-peridol, which decreases norepinephrine levels and more readily induces untoward effects such as sedation, depression, impaired motivation, cognitive dulling, irritability, phobias, and dyspho-ria, limiting the use of higher doses of haloperidol (Shapiro et al., 1983).

Investigational Reports of Interest

Shapiro and Shapiro (1984) performed a double-blind pla-cebo-controlled study of pimozide in 20 patients (mean age, 24.65 ± 2.71 years; range, 11 to 53 years) diagnosed with Tourette's syndrome. Six patients had a concomitant diagnosis of ADDH. The study was 14 weeks long—2 drug-free weeks followed by 6 weeks of one condition and then 6 weeks of the other. Initial dose of pimozide was 1 mg/day at bedtime, and dosage was flexibly adjusted every 2 to 3 days over 6 weeks to a maximum of 10 mg/day (approximately 0.2 mg/kg/day) for children and 20 mg/day for adults. Average optimal dose for pimozide was 6.88 ± 1.26 mg/day. The authors noted that effective dosage was relatively inde-pendent of age and that younger patients often required higher dosages than adults. Benztropine was used in 18 patients at some time during treatment to counteract extrapyramidal and akinesic effects. Pimozide was significantly more clinically effective (most measures at the $P = .0001$ level) than placebo on multiple de-pendent measures. The untoward effects of pimozide were similar to those of other high-potency antipsychotic drugs but were mostly of only slight to moderate intensity, an advantage over haloperidol (Shapiro & Shapiro, 1984).

Pangalila-Ratulangi (1973) reported a pilot study in which eight boys and two girls aged 9 to 14 years, eight of whom were diagnosed with schizophrenia or schizophrenia-like symptoms and two of whom had symptoms suggestive of epilepsy and blunted affect, improved clinically on doses of 1 to 2 mg/day of pimozide.

Naruse and colleagues (1982) assigned 87 children and ado-lescents aged 3 to 16 years randomly to haloperidol, pimozide, or placebo in a cross-over double-blind study. The subjects were diagnosed with various behavioral disorders, and 34 were autis-tic. Global ratings found pimozide to be clinically as effective as haloperidol and both to be superior to placebo. Pimozide, how-ever, was more clinically efficacious than haloperidol on behav-ioral rating scales. Sleepiness was the most common untoward effect and occurred in 24% (20) of the subjects receiving pimozide and 23% (19) receiving haloperidol versus only 4% (3) receiving placebo. Insomnia was the next most common side effect, occurring in 4% (3) of subjects on pimozide, 5% (4) of subjects on haloperidol, and 11% (9) of subjects on placebo.

Clozapine (Clozaril)

Indications in Child and Adolescent Psychiatry
Clozapine, a new "atypical" antipsychotic drug, was approved by the FDA for marketing in the United States in late 1989. It is a dibenzodiazepine and seems to have minimal central antidopaminergic activity; the manufacturer reports that no confirmed cases of tardive dyskinesia have been reported in over 15 years of worldwide experience.

Because of the increased risk for serious and potentially life-threatening untoward effects that has been reported in patients receiving clozapine, its administration is appropriate only for severely dysfunctional patients with schizophrenia who have not responded satisfactorily to adequate trials of at least two other standard antipsychotic drugs, or who cannot tolerate the untoward effects present at therapeutic dose levels.

The manufacturer notes that safety and efficacy of clozapine have not been established in children under 16 years of age.

Dosage Schedule for Children and Adolescents
- Children and adolescents under 16 years of age: Not recommended.
- Adolescents at least 16 years of age: Initially a dose of 25 mg once or twice daily is recommended. The dose can be increased daily by 25 to 50 mg, if tolerated, to reach a target dose of 300 to 450 mg by 2 weeks' time. Subsequent dose increases of a maximum of 100 mg may be made once or twice weekly. Total daily dosage should not exceed 900 mg.

Dose Forms Available
- Tablets: 25 mg, 100 mg

Untoward Effects of Clozapine

Agranulocytosis is reported to occur in association with administration of clozapine in between 1% and 2% of patients; however, with weekly monitoring and discontinuation of treatment if white blood cell counts dropped significantly, all cases of agranulocytosis reported in the United States following clozapine administration have been reversible, and no fatalities have been reported. Administration of clozapine is also associated with an increased incidence of seizures that is apparently dose dependent. At doses below 300 mg/day, about 1% to 2% of patients develop seizures; at moderate doses of 300 to 599 mg/day, about 3% to 4% develop seizures; at high doses of 600 to 900 mg/day, about 5% of patients develop seizures.

Other untoward effects include adverse cardiovascular effects such as orthostatic hypertension, tachycardia, and ECG changes.

Because of the relatively high risk of patients developing agranulocytosis, at the present time in the United States clozapine is available only through Sandoz Pharmaceuticals' Clozaril Patient Management System, which monitors hematological functioning through weekly blood tests, at which time the medication for the following week is dispensed to the patient. At the present time, the cost is very high, estimated at $9000 per year ("Assembly Moves," 1990).

Investigational Report of Interest

Siefen and Remschmidt (1986) administered clozapine to 21 inpatients, 12 of whom were below 18 years of age (average age, 18.1 years). Their patients had an average of 2.4 inpatient hospitalizations and had been tried on an average of 2.8 different antipsychotics without adequate therapeutic response or with severe extrapyramidal effects. In addition, the authors considered it a risk that their patients' psychotic symptoms would become chronic before clozapine was administered.

Clozapine was administered over an average of 133 days. The average maximum dose was 415 mg/day (range, 225 to 800 mg/day) and the average maintenance dose was 363 mg/day (range, 150 to 800 mg/day). In addition, 11 of the 21 subjects were administered one or more other unidentified drugs during about half of the time they were receiving clozapine.

About 67% of symptoms that had been relatively resistant to previous treatment with antipsychotics disappeared or improved markedly in 11 (52%) of patients, and an additional 6 (29%) patients showed at least slight improvement in the same number of symptoms. Four patients, however, had no changes or worsening of over half of their psychopathological symptoms during clozapine therapy. Positive symptoms of schizophrenia improved more than negative symptoms. Specifically, improvements in incoherent/dissociative thinking, aggressiveness, hallucinations, agitation, ideas of reference, anxiety, inability to make decisions, psychomotor agitation, motivation toward achievement, impoverished and restricted thinking, and ambivalent behavior were reported. Symptoms such as lack of self-confidence, fear of failure, psychomotor retardation, irritability, slowed thinking, blunted affect, and unhappiness showed no improvement or deteriorated during treatment with clozapine (Siefen & Remschmidt, 1986).

The most frequent untoward effects observed early in treatment with clozapine were daytime sedation, dizziness, tachycardia, orthostatic hypotension, sleepiness, and increased salivation. No patients developed agranulocytosis, and the hematological changes that occurred in about 25% of patients were clinically insignificant and normalized during continued maintenance on clozapine.

Siefen and Remschmidt (1986) concluded that clozapine was a particularly useful addition to the drug armamentarium in treating adolescents who do not respond satisfactorily to treatment with standard antipsychotics. As prepubertal children diagnosed with schizophrenia differ from adolescents and adults diagnosed with schizophrenia on some significant parameters and frequently respond less satisfactorily to treatment with standard antipsychotics, specific investigations of clozapine will be necessary to determine its efficacy in this age group (Green & Deutsch, 1990).

Antidepressants

INTRODUCTION

At the present time the tricyclics are the antidepressants of foremost importance in the treatment of children and younger adolescents. Although other types of antidepressants are approved for treating older adolescents diagnosed with depressive disorders (e.g., amoxapine [Asendin], a dibenzoxazepine antidepressant approved for persons at least 16 years of age), their use is essentially as for adults, and they will not be reviewed herein. Exceptions are made for some interesting studies in children and adolescents of monoamine oxidase inhibitors (MAOIs), the newly approved drug fluoxetine hydrochloride (Prozac), and bupropion hydrochloride (Wellbutrin), which is chemically unrelated to other antidepressants.

TRICYCLIC ANTIDEPRESSANTS

The tricyclic antidepressants have FDA approval for the treatment of depression in persons with a minimum age of 12 years. Imipramine is additionally approved for the treatment of enuresis in persons at least 6 years of age. There is, however, a considerable body of literature suggesting that imipramine is effective in the treatment of attention deficit hyperactivity disorder, school phobia (separation anxiety disorder), disorders of sleep (sleep terror disorder and sleepwalking disorder), and some children with major depressive disorder who were treated on an open basis. Clomipramine, another tricyclic antidepressant, has been recently approved by the FDA to be advertised as effective in the treatment of obsessive-compulsive disorder in persons at least 10 years of age.

At the present time, there are no formal criteria for the prophylactic use of tricyclic antidepressants in children and adolescents. The risks versus the benefits of long-term use for prevention of recurrences of mood disorders in this age group have not yet been established, and such use must be based on the physician's clinical judgment (National Institute of Mental Health/National Institutes of Health Consensus Development Panel, 1985).

Pharmacokinetics of Tricyclic Antidepressants

There may be large interindividual variations in steady-state plasma levels of tricyclics and their metabolites, although intraindividual levels are usually reproducible and correlate linearly with dose. Preskorn and his coworkers reported that steady-state imipramine plus desipramine levels varied 22-fold (from 25 to 553 ng/ml) among 68 hospitalized children aged 6 to 14 years, who were prescribed a fixed daily dose of 75 mg of imipramine to treat major depression ($N = 48$) or enuresis ($N = 20$) (Preskorn et al., 1989a). About 5% of the population may be genetically predisposed to metabolize tricyclic antidepressants more slowly than the general populace. Potter and his colleagues (1982) found that about 5% of 47 subjects, including 32 enuretic boys aged 7 to 13 years, were deficient desipramine hydroxylators and that such subjects had two to four times the steady-state concentrations of either imipramine or desipramine per unit dose as the general population. Preskorn and his colleagues warned that persons who metabolize tricyclics slowly may develop central nervous system toxicity, which may be confused with worsening of depression, or severe cardiotoxicity on conventional doses of tricyclics, and that deaths have occurred (Preskorn et al., 1989b). Because of these variables, it is desirable to obtain plasma levels whenever possible to avoid treatment failures for subtherapeutic levels or possible toxic effects from excessive levels.

Table 5.1 summarizes the development of symptoms of central nervous system toxicity. Preskorn et al. (1989b) have urged that therapeutic drug monitoring of tricyclic antidepressants be considered a routine standard of care for patients receiving tricyclic antidepressants.

Withdrawal of Medication

Some children experience a flu-like withdrawal syndrome, with gastrointestinal symptoms including nausea, abdominal discomfort and pain, vomiting, headache, and fatigue. These symp-

Table 5.1.
Evolution of Central Nervous System Tricyclic Toxicity[a]

Affective Symptoms	Motor Symptoms	Psychotic Symptoms	Organic Symptoms
Mood	Tremor	Thought disorder	Disorientation
↓ Concentration	Ataxia	Hallucination	↓ Memory
Lethargy	Seizures[b]	Delusions	Agitation
Social withdrawal			Confusion

[a] From Preskorn SH, Jerkovich GS, Beber JH, Widener P. Therapeutic drug monitoring of tricyclic antidepressants: a standard of care issue. Psychopharmacol Bull 1989;25:281–284.
[b] Seizures typically occur late but can occur earlier in the evolution.

toms result from cholinergic rebound and may be considered a cholinergic overdrive phenomenon. Ryan (1990) noted that because of their rapid metabolism of tricyclics, some prepubertal children and younger adolescents may show daily withdrawal effects if they receive their entire daily tricyclic medication in one dose, and hence it may be necessary to divide the medication into two or three doses.

When maintenance medication is discontinued, tapering the medication down over 10 days to 2 weeks rather than abruptly withdrawing the medication will usually avoid the development of a clinically significant withdrawal syndrome. The clinician is cautioned that in patients with poor compliance, who in essence may undergo periodic self-induced acute withdrawals, the resulting withdrawal syndrome may be confused with untoward effects of the medication, inadequate treatment, or worsening of the underlying condition.

Contraindications for Tricyclic Antidepressant Administration

Known hypersensitivity to tricyclic antidepressants is an absolute contraindication.

Tricyclic antidepressants are contraindicated for children and adolescents with cardiac conduction abnormalities.

Tricyclic antidepressants should not be administered concomitantly with an MAIO. At least a 14-day period must elapse after discontinuing an MAOI before administering a tricyclic antidepressant.

Tricyclics may lower the seizure threshold and should be used with caution in individuals with seizure disorder.

Tricyclic antidepressants may activate psychotic processes in schizophrenic patients.

Interactions of Tricyclic Antidepressants with Other Drugs

Hyperpyretic crises or severe convulsive seizures may occur in patient receiving MAOIs and tricyclic antidepressants simultaneously.

Anticholinergic effects of tricyclic antidepressants may be additive with those of antipsychotics and result in central nervous system anticholinergic toxicity.

The central nervous system depressive effects of tricyclic antidepressants may be additive with those of alcohol, benzodiazepines, barbiturates, and antipsychotics.

Tricyclic antidepressants may diminish or reverse the efficacy of antihypertensive agents.

Cigarette smoking may decrease the efficacy of tricyclic antidepressants.

Many other interactions with various drugs have also been reported.

Untoward Effects of Tricyclic Antidepressants

Cardiovascular side effects are of concern in all age groups but especially in children and younger adolescents. This is because children may be particularly vulnerable because of the relative efficiency with which they convert tricyclic antidepressants to potentially cardiotoxic 2-OH metabolites and children's being more sensitive to cardiotoxic effects that adolescents and adults (Baldessarini, 1990). Of particular concern are slowing of cardiac conduction as reflected on the ECG by increases in P-R and QRS intervals, cardiac arrhythmias, tachycardia, and heart block. Dugas and his colleagues (1980) have recommended that to avoid or minimize untoward effects related to peak serum levels, it is preferable to administer children tricyclic antidepressants two or three times daily if total doses are over 1 mg/kg, rather than to administer the total daily dose all at one time.

At least four sudden deaths have been reported in children taking tricyclic antidepressants, although these have not been proven to be cardiac related. A 6-year-old girl taking imipramine for chronic school phobia and separation anxiety died 3 days after the dose had been raised to 300 mg (14.7 mg/kg) at bedtime (Saraf et al., 1974). Sudden deaths were also reported in three boys treated with desipramine ("Sudden death," 1990). These were two 8-year-old boys diagnosed with ADD (one received desipramine for 2 years at an unknown dose, and one received the same drug for 6 months at 50 mg/day) and a 9-year-old boy whose diagnosis, dose, and duration of desipramine administration were not reported. All three of the boys had plasma levels in the therapeutic or subtherapeutic ranges ("Sudden Death," 1990).

Ryan and his colleagues (1987) reported that imipramine could safely be administered to adolescents in a single nighttime dose once dosage was stabilized, without significantly increased risk of heart block or other cardiovascular untoward effects. One advantage of giving the total dose at nighttime is that maximal sedative and anticholinergic untoward effects occur during sleep. The authors emphasized that their findings did not apply to prepubertal children who metabolize tricyclics more rapidly than adolescents and who may also be more sensitive to cardiotoxic effects (Ryan et al., 1987).

Central nervous system untoward effects may include drowsiness, EEG changes, seizures, incoordination, anxiety, insomnia and nightmares, confusion secondary to anticholinergic toxicity, delusions, and worsening of psychosis.

Tricyclic antidepressants may cause blood dyscrasias; if patients develop fever and sore throats during treatment with tricyclics, a CBC should be performed.

Anticholinergic untoward effects may include dry mouth, blurred vision, and constipation.

Changes in libido, both increases and decreases, have been reported; gynecomastia and impotence have also been reported.

Preskorn et al. (1988) reported that cognitive toxicity was associated with supratherapeutic plasma levels of tricyclics.

Tricyclic antidepressants, including clomipramine, may cause acute psychotic episodes if inadvertently administered to individuals with schizophrenia who have been incorrectly diagnosed.

TRICYCLIC ANTIDEPRESSANTS IN CHILD AND ADOLESCENT PSYCHIATRY

Imipramine Hydrochloride (Tofranil), Imipramine Pamoate (Tofranil-PM)

Because imipramine has been the most widely used clinically and has been more thoroughly studied in children and adolescents than the other tricyclics, it will serve as the prototype.

Indications in Child and Adolescent Psychiatry
    Imipramine is approved for use in treating symptoms of depression
in adolescents and adults. Its use in children is restricted to the treatment of enuresis in children who are at least 6 years old. Manufacturers
state that a maximum dose of 2.5 mg/kg should not be exceeded in
children (PDR, 1990).

Dosage Schedule for Children and Adolescents
• For Treating Depression:
    Children under 12 years of age: Not recommended (see, however, the
    reviews below of imipramine's use in this age group). Children at least
    12 years of age and adolescents: An initial dosage of 30 to 40 mg with
    gradual titration upward is suggested. It is generally not necessary to
    exceed 100 mg/day (manufacturer's package insert) (see, however,
    the discussion below on treating adolescents and the importance of
    determining serum levels).
• For Treating Enuresis:
    Recommended dosages differ from those for depression and are
    given below in the section "Impramine in the Treatment of Enuresis."
• For Attention Deficit Hyperactivity Disorder:
    Recommended dosages are given below in the section "Imipramine
    in the Treatment of Attention Deficit Hyperactivity Disorder."

Dose Forms Available
• Tablets (imipramine hydrochloride): 10 mg, 25 mg, 50 mg
• Capsules (imipramine pamoate): 75 mg, 100 mg, 125 mg, 150 mg
    (These capsules are designed for once-daily dosing. Because of their
    high unit potency and the greater sensitivity of children to the cardio-
    toxic effects of imipramine, their use is not recommended in children
    and younger adolescents.)

Untoward Effects of Imipramine

Imipramine has many untoward effects, some of which are
potentially life threatening. Cardiovascular effects, including arrhythmias, tachycardia, blood pressure changes, impaired conduction and heart block, and a decreased seizure threshold, are
particularly worrisome. See also the section "Untoward Effects of
Tricyclic Antidepressants," above.

Imipramine in the Treatment of Enuresis

Although the pharmacological treatment of enuresis has been
shown to be effective (Poussaint & Ditman, 1965; Rapoport et al.,
1980b), it should not be employed until possible organic etiologies
have been ruled out by appropriate physical examination and
tests. It should be emphasized that behavioral therapies (e.g.,

conditioning with a bell and pad apparatus) are the treatments of choice for functional enuresis. There is a tendency for some children to become tolerant of imipramine's antienuretic effects, and many children relapse after medication withdrawal.

Imipramine's antienuretic effect occurs rapidly and appears to be unrelated to its antidepressant effects; it may directly inhibit bladder musculature and increase outlet resistance (American Medical Association, 1986). It also appears that the imipramine plus desipramine plasma level required for the effective treatment of enuresis is lower than that required for treating major depressive disorder. DeGatta et al. (1984) treated 90 enuretic patients aged 5 to 14 years with imipramine and reported that the minimum efficient serum concentration of imipramine plus desipramine in most cases was 80 ng/ml. However, about 20% of the subjects did not respond satisfactorily to imipramine even with adequate serum levels.

A trial of imipramine may occasionally be indicated when safer and more efficacious methods have failed and the symptom is psychologically handicapping or distressing to the patient, or, perhaps, when rapid control is essential to permit a child to go to summer camp or travel.

The most frequent untoward effects reported in the treatment of enuretic children with imipramine are nervousness, sleep disorders, tiredness, and mild gastrointestinal disturbances (PDR, 1990). DeGatta et al. (1984) reported that 40% of their 90 enuretic subjects had at least one side effect; 42% had loss of appetite, 16% had light sleep, 11% had abdominal pains, 8% had dry mouth, and 8% had headaches.

In clinical practice, initial ECGs are not usually done for the treatment of enuresis, as the final total daily dosage of imipramine usually remains below 2.5 mg/kg and risk of cardiotoxicity is low. It is suggested that bedwetters who void soon after falling asleep benefit if imipramine is given earlier and in divided doses (e.g., 25 mg in midafternoon and 25 mg before bed) (PDR, 1990).

Dosage Schedule for Treating Enuresis
- Children under 6 years of age: Not recommended.
- Children at least 6 years of age through 11 years: Begin with 25 mg 1 hour before bedtime. If not effective within 1 week, increase to maximum dose of 50 mg.
- Persons at least 12 years of age: Proceed as above, with the option to increase the dose to a maximum of 75 mg.

Investigational Reports of Interest

Imipramine in the Treatment of Childhood (Prepubertal) Major Depressive Disorder

It is well established that prepubertal children can be diagnosed with major depressive disorder (MDD) using research diagnostic criteria (RDC) (Spitzer et al., 1978) or DSM-III (APA, 1980a) criteria (Puig-Antich, 1987). A literature review of the use of tricyclic antidepressants in children and adolescents with major depression found them to be clinically effective in several open studies, but no double-blind placebo-controlled study reported that tricyclics were superior to placebo (Ambrosini, 1987).

At the present time, imipramine and nortriptyline are the only tricyclics approved by the FDA for investigational use for depression in children aged 12 years and under. Current FDA guidelines for ECG changes during treatment with either drug are as follows:

1. The P-R interval should not exceed 0.21 second.
2. Resting heart rate should be less than 130 beats per minute.
3. The QRS interval should not exceed 0.02 seconds more than the baseline interval.

The blood pressure of children receiving imipramine, which can both elevate the blood pressure and produce orthostatic hypotension, should not be permitted to exceed 145/95 mm Hg (Geller & Carr, 1988). Imipramine levels above 5 mg/kg are not usually permitted in investigational protocols (Hayes et al., 1975).

Baseline studies that should be completed before initiating treatment with a tricyclic antidepressant include sitting and supine blood pressure, complete blood count (CBC) with differential, electrolytes, thyroid function tests, blood urea nitrogen (BUN), serum creatinine, urinalysis with osmolality, liver function tests, and an ECG. Many clinicians do not do an ECG if using imipramine in the low doses recommended for enuresis (a maximum of 75 mg/day).

Several investigators have noted that in clinical practice an absolute upper dose maximum for tricyclic antidepressants is not very useful because of the marked intersubject variability in pharmacokinetics (e.g., metabolism and elimination) and the fact that although children as a group tend to metabolize and/or eliminate tricyclic antidepressants more rapidly than older adolescents and adults, some children, perhaps genetically slow hydroxylators, may reach very high serum levels on doses well below the recommended maximum (Biederman et al., 1989b). Hence careful clinical monitoring, including serum levels if available, is essential.

Puig-Antich and his colleagues (1987) investigated the use of imipramine in prepubescent children diagnosed with MDD. In a double-blind placebo-controlled study of 38 subjects, there was no significant difference between response to imipramine (56%; 9 of 16 subjects) and response to placebo (68%; 15 of 22 subjects).

These authors also studied total maintenance plasma level (imipramine plus desipramine) in 30 prepubescent children and found a positive correlation between plasma level and clinical response. Responders had significantly higher ($P < .007$) mean maintenance total plasma levels (284 ± 225 ng/ml) than did nonresponders (145 ± 80 ng/ml). The authors reported that a maintenance total plasma level of 150 ng/ml was the most important differentiating point between responders and nonresponders. Eighty-five percent of subjects (17 of 20) whose values were above 150 ng/ml had positive responses, but only 30% (3 of 10) of children with lower values responded positively. The authors also found nothing, including dosage, that predicted plasma levels (Puig-Antich et al., 1987). This is consonant with the finding that combined imipramine and desipramine steady-state plasma levels varied sixfold (from 56 to 324 ng/ml) in 11 boys receiving 75 mg/day of imipramine (Weller et al., 1982).

Other important findings of Puig-Antich and his colleagues (1987) were (a) the more severe the pretreatment depressive symptoms on the K-SADS nine-item depressive score, the less likely was a favorable response to imipramine ($P < .008$); (b) prepubescent children with the RDC psychotic subtype of MDD were much less likely to have a favorable response to imipramine than nonpsychotic depressed children ($P < .05$); and (c) some children would require dosages over 5 mg/kg/day to reach plasma levels in the range associated with positive response.

These authors also reported that the following untoward effects were found in over 30% of the children treated with imipramine: excitement, irritability, nightmares, insomnia, headache, muscle pain, increased appetite, abdominal cramps, constipation, vomiting, hiccups, dry mouth, bad taste in the mouth, sweating, flushed face, drowsiness, dizziness, tiredness, and restlessness. Similar untoward effects were present in the placebo group, although at lower frequencies. The untoward effects were severe enough in 17 of the 30 children to prevent upward titration to 5 mg/kg/day; cardiac side effects were responsible in 10 of these cases. Nine children had increases in the P-R interval to the maximum, and one child's resting heart rate reached 130 beats per minute. No child on placebo showed ECG changes from baseline, whereas nearly every child receiving imipramine had at least minor changes (Puig-Antich et al., 1987).

Based on their own data and that of Puig-Antich and his coworkers, Preskorn et al. (1989a) concluded that plasma imipramine plus desipramine levels ranging from 125 to 250 ng/ml were both efficacious and safe in treating MDD in children. These authors suggested using an initial oral dose of 75 mg imipramine daily and then determining the combined plasma concentration of imipramine plus desipramine 7 to 10 days later when steady-state levels would be expected. Based on their experience, 78% of children initially had plasma levels outside the therapeutic range; 66% were below 125 ng/ml, and 12% were above 250 ng/ml. As intraindividual plasma levels were reproducible and linearly correlated with dose, the authors used a formula, new dose = (initial dose/initial level) × desired level, to adjust the dosage. Desired level was 185 ng/ml, the midpoint of the optimal range. Using this strategy, 84% of their patients achieved levels within the therapeutic range. The remaining 16% had subtherapeutic levels, possibly requiring additional adjustments (Preskorn et al., 1989a).

Imipramine in the Treatment of Adolescent Major Depressive Disorder

Thirty-four adolescents with MDD treated with imipramine in an open study with monitoring of plasma imipramine levels showed some differences from prepubescent children (Ryan et al., 1986). Imipramine was titrated to a dose of 5 mg/kg/day; the adolescents had an overall positive response rate of 44% (15 of 34), but there was no relationship between positive response and higher plasma imipramine levels. Another difference between the adolescents and prepubertal children with MDD was that as a group, nonpsychotic subjects did not respond more favorably than the psychotic subtype. The authors hypothesized that adolescents with MDD were less responsive to imipramine because of an antagonistic effect of sex hormones, levels of which increase during adolescence (Ryan et al., 1986).

Strober et al. (1990) treated openly with imipramine 35 adolescents aged 13 years to 18 years of age (mean, 15.4 years) who were hospitalized and diagnosed by RDC criteria with MDD with at least probable certainty, 10 of whom also met criteria for delusional subtype. After failing to improve after a week's hospitalization, subjects were treated for 6 weeks with imipramine. Only 6 of the 34 subjects who completed the study were unable to achieve the target dose of 5 mg/kg/day, because of untoward effects. Average daily dose was 222 ± 49 mg/day, and steady-state imipramine plus desmethylimipramine levels varied 11-fold (mean, 237 ± 168 ng/ml; range, 79 to 888 ng/ml). Only eight (33%) of the nondelusional subjects and 1 (10%) of the delusional subjects were considered responders, suggesting greater refractoriness in patients with psychotic features. No responders had a plasma imipramine plus desmethylimipramine level below 180 ng/ml, but the difference between responders and nonresponders was not significant. Overall, only 10 (29.4%) patients were rated very much improved or much improved on the Clinical Global Impressions Improvement scale.

Ryan et al. (1988a) treated 14 adolescents aged 14 to 19 years (mean, 16.9 years) who were diagnosed by RDC with nonbipolar MDD and who had not responded to treatment with various tricyclic antidepressants (for a period of at least 6 weeks in 12 cases and for 4 weeks in 2 cases) by augmenting their treatment with lithium while continuing treatment with amitriptyline, desipramine, or nortriptyline. Lithium carbonate was titrated to achieve therapeutic serum levels. Six patients (43%) were responders and improved to the extent of having at most mild symptoms of depression and were no longer being functionally impaired by their depression. Most responders improved gradually over the 1st month after the addition of lithium treatment. Their serum lithium level was 0.65 ± 0.06 mEq/liter and was not significantly different from that of the nonresponders. The authors suggested that the addition of lithium carbonate may be a useful adjunct to the treatment of some adolescents with major depression who do not respond satisfactorily to treatment with tricyclic antidepressants (Ryan et al., 1988a).

Imipramine in the Treatment of Attention Deficit Hyperactivity Disorder

There is a considerable literature attesting to the clinical efficacy of imipramine in the treatment of attention deficit hyperactivity disorder (ADHD), although most studies find stimulants superior (for review see Campbell et al., 1985; Rapoport & Mikkelsen, 1978, Rapoport et al., 1974). Although imipramine does not have FDA approval for use in ADHD, some clinicians consider imipramine the next drug of choice if a patient does not respond to stimulants. Wender (1988), however, notes that when used to treat ADHD, tricyclics improve mood and decrease hyperactivity but usually are sedating and do not appear to improve concentration.

The mechanism of action of imipramine in ADHD is different from that in depression; it is rapidly effective, and often lower doses are required. Mean dosages reported in the literature have ranged from 20 to 173.7 mg/day. The development of tolerance by some children to the therapeutic effects of imipramine within about 6 weeks presents difficulties.

Dosage Schedule for Treating ADHD
- No official recommendations for age or dose exist. Based on the literature and experimental protocols, the following is suggested for children over 6 years of age. Monitoring prerequisites for imipramine should be followed. Begin with a low dose, either 25 mg/day or 0.5 mg/kg/day, and slowly titrate upward with increases of 25 mg once or twice weekly.

Imipramine in the Treatment of Separation Anxiety Disorder (School Phobia)

Imipramine has been used with some success in treating school-phobic children (for review see Klein et al., 1980, pp. 712–718). Klein et al. (1980) emphasize that imipramine is effective in reducing separation anxiety but that anticipatory anxiety may continue to be problematic. Imipramine doses of between 75 and 200 mg/day were effective for school-phobic children between 6 and 14 years of age; however, children with severe separation anxiety without school phobia sometimes responded to doses as low as 25 to 50 mg/day (Klein et al., 1980).

School-phobic children who responded to imipramine were found to show at least some improvement when doses reached 125 mg/day; once improvement began, further dose increases usually produced additional benefit. Response was usually maximal within 6 to 8 weeks. It was suggested that maintenance be continued for a minimum of 8 weeks following remission of symptoms and then tapered and discontinued (Klein et al., 1980).

Recently, it was reported that three children with panic disorder who also had severe separation anxiety and agoraphobia responded well to a combination of imipramine and alprazolam, a benzodiazepine (Ballenger et al., 1989).

Imipramine in the Treatment of Somnambulism and Night Terrors

Four children with night terrors, two children with somnambulism, and one child with both disorders were treated with imipramine (10 to 50 mg at bedtime). The sleep disorders remitted completely in all children (Pesikoff & Davis, 1971).

Nortriptyline Hydrochloride (Pamelor)

Indications in Child and Adolescent Psychiatry
Nortriptyline is approved by the FDA for the treatment of symptoms of depression in adolescents and adults. The drug is not recommended for use in the pediatric age group as its safety and effectiveness have not been established in children.

Dosage Schedule for Children and Adolescents
- Children: Not recommended.
- Adolescents: Manufacturer recommends giving a total of 30 to 50 mg/ day. One should start at a low dose and titrate upward based on clinical response. (See, however, recommendations of Geller and her colleagues below on the usefulness of serum levels.)

Dose Forms Available
- Capsules: 10 mg, 25 mg, 50 mg, 75 mg
- Oral solution: 10 mg/5 ml

Untoward effects of the tricyclic antidepressants are discussed above in "Untoward Effects of Tricyclic Antidepressants," as well as in the summary of the work of Geller and her colleagues, below.

Investigational Reports of Interest

Nortriptyline in the Treatment of Major Depressive Disorder in Children and Adolescents

Geller and her colleagues have studied pharmacokinetic parameters of nortriptyline and its use in treating in children and adolescents diagnosed with major depressive disorder (MDD) (Geller et al., 1986, 1987b, 1989, 1990). There are no double-blind placebo-controlled studies establishing nortriptyline's superiority over placebo in treating MDD in children or adolescents.

Nortriptyline in the Treatment of Depressed Children

In an open study, Geller et al. (1986) found that therapeutic efficacy correlated with nortriptyline plasma levels. Twenty-two children 6 to 12 years old diagnosed with MDD were treated on an outpatient basis with fixed doses of either 10 mg twice daily or 25 mg twice daily for 8 weeks. Initial dose was based on individual subjects' rate of metabolism of nortriptyline, as determined by baseline single-dose kinetics, with the slower metabolizers receiving the lower fixed dose. Fourteen subjects (63.6%) responded favorably to nortriptyline. Responders were not significantly different from nonresponders in terms of age, sex, weight, social class, duration of illness, or baseline or 2-week Children's Depression Rating Scale scores. Responders, however, had significantly higher mean mg/kg daily doses (1.02 ± 0.21 mg/kg; range, 0.64 to 1.57 mg/kg) than nonresponders (0.82 ± 0.51 mg/kg; range, 0.40 to 2.01 mg/kg). The mean nortriptyline steady-state plasma level was also higher in responders (60.31 ± 20.90 ng/ml; range, 18.8 to 111.5 ng/ml)) than in nonresponders (30.86 ± 17.64 ng/ml; range, 12 to 54.3 ng/ml). Twelve of the 13 subjects who received at least 0.89 mg/kg/day responded. All subjects with steady-state nortriptyline plasma levels of at least 60 ng/ml responded, as did 4 of 7 children with levels ranging from 40 to 59 ng/ml. At the end of the 8-week protocol, 7 of the 8 nonresponders recovered when nortriptyline dose was increased to achieve steady-state nortriptyline plasma levels of 60 to 100 ng/ml. Overall, 21 of the 22 subjects had good clinical response with minimal and transient side effects, and all ECGs remained within recommended parameters for prepubertal children. These authors felt that since children's plasma nortriptyline levels are stable over time, ECGs need to be performed only at baseline and once at steady-state plasma levels if they remain within recommended parameters (Geller et al., 1986).

Geller and her colleagues (1989) enrolled 72 prepubescent children aged 6 years to 12 years who were diagnosed with MDD, nondelusional type, by Research Diagnostic Criteria (RDC) (Spitzer et al., 1978) and DSM-III (1980) criteria in a double-blind placebo-controlled study of the efficacy of nortriptyline. The study design was a 2-week single-blind placebo washout phase followed by an 8-week random assignment double-blind placebo-controlled phase. All subjects were outpatients, and most had coexisting separation anxiety. The children were chronically depressed: 96% had been ill for at least 2 years, and 50% had had

MDD for 5 or more years before entering the study. Of the 72 subjects entering the study, 12 (16.7%) responded during the placebo phase, 10 were discontinued for various reasons during the active treatment phase, and 50 (24 on placebo and 26 on nortriptyline) completed the study.

Using a table (see below), the initial dose necessary to achieve a steady-state nortriptyline level of 80 ± 20 ng/ml was determined from 24-hour plasma levels. Any necessary adjustments to obtain mean steady-state plasma levels of nortriptyline and of total, trans, and cis 10-hydroxynortriptyline (10-OH-NT) were made during the first 4 weeks of the double-blind phase.

Both the nortriptyline and the placebo groups had a low rate of positive response (30.8% on nortriptyline and 16.7% on placebo), and there was no significant difference between them. There was no significant correlation between mean nortriptyline plasma level and response, or between mean nortriptyline plus mean total, cis, or trans 10-OH-NT plasma levels and response. Because of the poor response rate and the unlikelihood of finding a statistical difference between the placebo and active groups if the protocol were completed, Geller et al. (1989) stopped their study at this point.

Nortriptyline in the Treatment of Depressed Adolescents

Geller et al. (1990) enrolled 52 postpubertal adolescents aged 12 to 17 years with RDC (Spitzer et al., 1978) and DSM-III (1980a) MDD in a random assignment double-blind placebo-controlled study of nortriptyline. Adolescents with delusional symptoms were not enrolled. Subjects had scores on the Children's Depression Rating Scale (CDRS) and the Kiddie Global Assessment Scale (KGAS) placing them in the severe range of pathology. Of the 31 subjects completing the study, 27 (87.1%) of subjects had a duration of symptoms for at least 2 years: 10 (32.3%) between 2 and 5 years and 17 (54.8%) more than 5 years.

The study was comprised of a 2-week single-blind placebo washout phase and an 8-week double-blind placebo-controlled phase. Using a table (see below), initial dose necessary to achieve a steady-state nortriptyline level of 80 ± 20 ng/ml was determined from 24-hour plasma levels. Mean nortriptyline plasma level was 91.1 ± 18.3 ng/ml.

Of the 52 subjects enrolled, 17 (32.7%) responded to placebo by the end of week 2, and 4 additional subjects dropped out for other reasons. Of the 31 completing the study, 12 were assigned to nortriptyline and 19 to placebo. The results of the study showed such a low rate of response to nortriptyline that the study was terminated early. Only 1 (8.3%) of 12 subjects receiving nortriptyline responded, while 4 (21.1%) of the 19 subjects on placebo responded. (The one responder to nortriptyline went on to have a bipolar course.) Subjects with higher nortriptyline levels achieved significantly worse scores on the CDRS ($P = .002$). There were, however, no significant differences between the two groups on final CDRS or KGAS scores.

It is most interesting that 17, or about one-third of enrolled patients, with chronic and severe depression responded to placebo within 2 weeks. However, 13 of the 17 placebo responders relapsed, 9 of them within 1 to 4 weeks (Geller et al., 1990).

Nortriptyline Dosage Schedule for Children and Adolescents

Pharmacokinetic studies of tricyclic antidepressants in adults have shown that their elimination half-lives are sufficiently long to permit the frequent practice of giving a single bedtime dose once titration is completed (Rudorfer & Potter, 1987). Geller et al. (1987b), however, note that 41 children 5 to 12 years old had a significantly shorter mean nortriptyline plasma half-life (20.8 ± 7.2 hours; range, 11.2 to 42.5 hours) than 32 adolescents 13 to 16 years old (31.1 ± 19.8 hours; range, 14.2 to 76.6 hours). Geller et al. (1985) also found that correlations between the milligram per kilogram dose of nortriptyline and steady-state plasma levels were not significant in 33 children and adolescents 5 to 16 years of age. The clinical significance of these data, including the interindividual variation of half-life by as much as six- or sevenfold, prompted Geller et al. (1987b) to advise that nortriptyline should be administered twice daily for all patients up through 16 years of age and that plasma level monitoring is essential to be sure of achieving therapeutic plasma nortriptyline levels.

Geller et al. (1985) have used a single test dose of nortriptyline to predict steady-state plasma levels and to determine the initial dose of nortriptyline and presented tables suggesting daily doses to reach therapeutic nortriptyline plasma levels (see Table 5.2). To use this method, the clinician must have access to a laboratory that can reliably assay nortriptyline levels of less than 20 ng/ml.

To use this table clinically, Geller et al. (1985) and Geller and Carr (1988) suggested the following:

1. At 9:00 A.M. administer a single dose of 25 mg to patients 5 to 9 years of age, or 50 mg to patients 10 to 16 years of age.

Table 5.2.
Suggested Nortriptyline Dose Schedules for Children and Adolescents[a]

Predicted doses from 24-hour plasma levels after a single dose of 25 mg administered to 5- to 9-year-olds.[b]	
24-hour plasma level (ng/mg)	Suggested total daily dose (mg)
6–10	50–75
11–14	35–40
15–20	25–30
21–25	20
Predicted doses from 24-hour nortriptyline plasma levels after a single dose of 50 mg administered to 10- to 16-year-olds.[b]	
24-hour plasma level (ng/mg)	Suggested total daily dose (mg)
10–14	75–100
15–19	50–75
20–24	40–50
25–29	35
30–34	30
35–40	25
>40	20

[a] Adapted from Geller B, Cooper TB, Chestnut EC, et al. Child and adolescent nortriptyline single dose kinetics predict steady state plasma levels and suggested dose: preliminary data. J Clin Psychopharmacol 1985;5:154–158.
[b] Total daily dose should be divided and given twice daily because of relatively short half-life.

2. Twenty-four hours later (9:00 A.M. the next day) draw blood to determine the plasma nortriptyline level.
3. Use the table to determine the suggested medication dose for the patient's nortriptyline level and age.
4. Seven days later determine plasma nortriptyline level 9 to 11 hours after a dose. If level is not in the therapeutic range (60 to 100 ng/ml), adjust the dosage using the following formula (Geller & Carr, 1988):

$$\frac{\text{Day 7 plasma level}}{\text{Current dose}} = \frac{80 \text{ ng/ml}}{\text{Adjusted dose}}$$

Geller et al. (1987b) have recommended that nortriptyline be withdrawn gradually over approximately 10 days to 2 weeks, to avoid withdrawal symptoms. Only 6 of 30 children and adolescents 6 to 16 years old developed withdrawal symptoms when this was done. In all cases symptoms were mild, and in 5 subjects they were limited to the gastrointestinal system and consisted of stomachache, nausea, and/or emesis.

Amitriptyline Hydrochloride (Elavil, Endep)

Indications in Child and Adolescent Psychiatry
Amitriptyline is approved to treat symptoms of depression. It is noted that endogenous depression is more likely to be alleviated than are other depressive states. It is not recommended for patients under 12 years of age because of limited experience with treating this age group with amitriptyline.

Dosage Schedule in Children and Adolescents
- Children under 12 years of age: Not recommended.
- Children and adolescents at least 12 years old: Ten milligrams three times daily and 20 mg at bedtime may be adequate for adolescents who do not tolerate higher doses. The usual maintenance dose is 50 to 100 mg/day. An initial dose of 25 mg/day titrated upward in 25 mg increments is suggested.

Dose Forms Available
- Tablets: 10 mg, 25 mg, 50 mg, 75 mg, 100 mg
- Injectable: 10 mg/ml

Untoward effects of amitriptyline are discussed above in "Untoward Effects of Tricyclic Antidepressants."

Investigational Reports of Interest

Amitriptyline in Depressed Children

Kashani et al. (1984) performed a double-blind cross-over study comparing amitriptyline and placebo in nine prepubertal depressed children. Dosage ranged from 45 to 110 mg/day. Six (66.7%) of the subjects improved on amitriptyline, which was not significant ($P < .09$).

Amitriptyline in Depressed Adolescents

Kramer and Feiguine (1981) compared the efficacy of amitriptyline and placebo in treating 20 adolescents diagnosed with depression. Age range was 13 to 17 years. Amitriptyline was initially given in 25-mg doses four times daily and increased within 3 days to a maximum of 200 mg/day in divided doses. The length of the study was 6 weeks. Both placebo and active medication groups improved over the 6-week period, and there was no significant difference between the two groups. Although this pilot study suggests that amitriptyline is no more effective than placebo in treating adolescent depression, more studies and larger numbers are necessary before definitively concluding this.

Desipramine Hydrochloride (Norpramine, Pertofrane)

Indications in Child and Adolescent Psychiatry
   Desipramine is indicated in the treatment of symptoms in various depressive syndromes, especially endogenous depression. Its efficacy and safety have not been established for children.

Dosage Schedule for Children and Adolescents
- Children: Not recommended.
- Adolescents: Usual dose is between 25 and 100 mg/day. One should start at a lower dose and titrate according to clinical response. A dose of 150 mg/day should not be exceeded. Adequate treatment response may take 2 to 3 weeks to develop.

Dose Forms Available
- Tablets: 10 mg, 25 mg, 50 mg, 75 mg, 100 mg, 150 mg

Untoward effects of the tricyclics, including sudden death with desipramine, are discussed above in "Untoward Effects of the Tricyclic Antidepressants."

Investigational Reports of Interest

Desipramine in the Treatment of Enuresis

Rapoport et al. (1980b) found that 75 mg of desipramine at bedtime had a short-term antienuretic effect that was not statistically different from that of imipramine.

Desipramine in the Treatment of ADHD

Garfinkel et al. (1983) studied 12 males (mean age, 7.3 years; range, 5.9 to 11.6 years) who were diagnosed with attention deficit disorder and required day hospital or inpatient treatment for the severity of their symptoms of impulsiveness, inattention, and aggression. The subjects received placebo, methylphenidate, desipramine, and clomipramine in a double-blind cross-over experiment. Mean dose of desipramine was 85 mg/day and did not exceed 100 mg/day or 3.5 mg/kg/day for any subject. Methylphenidate was significantly better than the other three conditions in improving overall classroom functioning as rated on the Conners Scale by teachers ($P < .005$) and program child care workers ($P < .001$).

Biederman et al. (1989a, 1989b) reviewed earlier work in this area and studied the efficacy of desipramine in treating 42 children and 20 adolescents diagnosed with attention deficit disorder with hyperactivity ($N = 60$) or without hyperactivity ($N = 2$).

Sixty-nine percent of their subjects had responded poorly to earlier treatment with stimulants. The subjects were randomly assigned to a 6-week, double-blind, parallel groups, placebo-controlled protocol. Desipramine was titrated upward to an average dose of 4.6 mg/kg ± 0.2 mg/kg, a relatively high dose. This high dose was selected because of inconsistent findings in studies using lower doses of desipramine in subjects with ADD (Biederman et al., 1989a). Patients treated with desipramine had statistically significant improvement in symptoms rated on the Conners Abbreviated Parent and Teacher Questionnaires, compared to subjects receiving placebo ($P = .0001$). The patterns of improvement were similar in adolescents and children. There was no significant relationship between serum desipramine levels and clinical response making the designation of an optimal level inappropriate. Some subjects who improved had serum levels below 100 ng/ml. About one-fourth of the patients had high levels, between 300 and 900 ng/ml; of this group 80% (12 of 15) improved (Biederman et al., 1989b).

Untoward effects were usually mild and were more frequent in subjects receiving desipramine than in the placebo group ($P < .05$); overall, there was no discernible relationship between serum level and untoward effects. Symptoms included dry mouth (32%), decreased appetite (29%), headache (29%), abdominal discomfort (26%), tiredness (25%), dizziness (23%), and insomnia (23%). Although no subjects developed any clinically apparent cardiovascular signs or symptoms, cardiovascular and ECG untoward effects, such as increased diastolic blood pressure, tachycardia, and conduction abnormalities, were statistically more frequent in subjects receiving desipramine. There was a suggestion that ECG changes occurred more frequently at higher serum desipramine levels. Although side effects were rated as mild, the authors noted that in 71% of patients (22 of 31) receiving desipramine and 52% of patients (16 of 31) receiving placebo, untoward effects prevented the medication from being raised to the target dose of 5 mg/kg/day (Biederman et al., 1989b). Of special interest is that in contrast to reports of rapid improvement of subjects with ADD in response to imipramine, subjects in this study required 3 to 4 weeks to show significant clinical improvement with desipramine as compared to placebo (Biederman et al., 1989b).

Schroeder et al. (1989) reported that the cardiovascular effects of desipramine in 20 children aged 7 years to 12 years who were treated with maximum doses of up to 5 mg/kg/day and an average of 4.25 mg/kg/day were a 21% increase in cardiac rate and a 2.5% increase in the Q-T interval. Arrhythmias and clinically meaningful blood pressure changes did not occur. The authors concluded that from a cardiotoxicity viewpoint, desipramine was safe in children without heart disease, although the ECG should be monitored appropriately (Schroeder et al., 1989).

Biederman et al. (1989b) suggested that a steady-state serum desipramine level between 100 ng/ml and a maximum of 300 ng/ml is probably efficacious and safe for most children and adolescents but that some patients will require daily doses greater than 3.5 mg/kg/day to reach these serum levels. They estimated that optimal doses range between 2.5 and 5 mg/kg/day. The authors (Biederman et al., 1989b) recommended that the following parameters are more clinically relevant in the titration of desipramine than accepting an arbitrary maximum limit in dose (e.g., 5 mg/kg):

1. The desipramine serum level should be kept under 300 ng/ml.
2. The P-R interval on the ECG should be less that 200 msec.
3. The QRS interval on the ECG should be less than 120 msec.

Desipramine shows some promise as an alternative medication for children and adolescents diagnosed with ADHD who have unsatisfactory responses to stimulant medication. Its use requires strict clinical monitoring, including ECG and serum levels, and must be considered investigational at the present time.

Desipramine in the Treatment of Coexisting ADHD and Tics

Although stimulants are the treatment of choice in ADHD, they may exacerbate tics or precipitate them *de novo*. Hence problems arise when children have preexisting tic disorders, or when they develop tics while being treated with stimulants. Indeed, some authorities recommend not giving stimulants to children with a family history of tics or Tourette's disorder.

Riddle and his colleagues (1988) noted that Tourette's disorder and ADHD coexist in approximately 50% of children who are referred for evaluation of Tourette's disorder and that between 20% and 50% of such patients develop worsening of their tics if treated with stimulants. The authors treated with desipramine seven children aged 7 years to 11 years, all of whom had diagnoses of ADHD and various tic disorders (one with Tourette's disorder, three with chronic multiple tics, and two with family histories of Tourette's disorder, four of whom had developed chronic tic symptoms when previously treated with methylphenidate); five of the children had an additional diagnosis of oppositional disorder. Desipramine was begun at 25 mg daily and increased by 25 mg every 2 to 3 days to a maximum of 100 mg, or a lower level when clinical improvement was satisfactory or untoward effects prevented further increase. Four children improved "remarkably" and one child "moderately" when rated on the Clinician's Global Improvement Scale; two children were considered nonresponders. Six children showed no change in the status or severity of their tics. One child's intermittent eyeblinking became persistent after 3 weeks of desipramine; this had also occurred in this patient during a previous trial of methylphenidate (Riddle et al., 1988).

Although further experience is necessary to establish that desipramine is both safe and efficacious in treating children and adolescents with coexisting ADHD and tic disorder, it appears to be a potentially useful alternative treatment for such children whose ADHD is of sufficient severity to necessitate pharmacological intervention and for those children diagnosed with ADHD who develop tics following the initiation of stimulant therapy.

Clomipramine Hydrochloride (Anafranil)

Clomipramine is an antiobsessional drug that belongs to the class of tricyclic antidepressants. Clomipramine itself has potent inhibitory effects on the neuronal reuptake of serotonin as compared to neuronal reuptake of norepinephrine; however, its primary metabolite, desmethylclomipramine, effectively inhibits norepinephrine uptake.

Flàment and colleagues (1987) studied the actions of clomipramine on peripheral measures of serotonergic and noradrenergic function in children and adolescents diagnosed with obsessive-compulsive disorder. They compared 29 such children and adolescents (mean age, 13.9 ± 2.5 years; range, 8 to 18 years) with controls and found that a high pretreatment level of platelet serotonin was a strong predictor of a favorable clinical response and that clomipramine treatment produced a very marked decrease in platelet serotonin concentration for all patients ($P <$ .0001). Clomipramine treatment also produced a trend toward reduction in platelet MAO activity ($P = .11$) and increased peripheral noradrenergic function. The plasma level of norepinephrine in standing subjects increased significantly ($P <$

.008). These data suggest that clomipramine's inhibition of serotonin uptake may be essential to its antiobsessional effect (Flament et al., 1987).

Indications in Child and Adolescent Psychiatry
Clomipramine has been recently been approved by the FDA for the treatment of obsessions and compulsions in patients at least 10 years of age who have been diagnosed with obsessive-compulsive disorder.

Dosage Schedule for Children and Adolescents
- Children under age 10: Not recommended.
- Children at least 10 years old and adolescents to 17 years of age: Initial dose of 25 mg/day, titrated upward to a daily maximum of 100 mg or 3 mg/kg/day, whichever is less, over the 1st 2 weeks. Subsequently dosage may be increased gradually to a maximum of 200 mg/day or 3 mg/kg/day, whichever is less. After the optimal dose has been determined, clomipramine may be given in a single bedtime dose to minimize daytime sedation.
- Adolescents at least 18 years old: As above, but maximum dose may be increased to 250 mg/day.
- Abrupt withdrawal of clomipramine may result in withdrawal symptoms similar to those that occur when the tricyclics used in treating depression are suddenly discontinued. Symptoms may include dizziness, nausea, vomiting, headache, malaise, sleep disturbances, hyperthermia, irritability, and worsening of psychiatric status. Hence a gradual tapering of the dose over a period of 10 days to 2 weeks is recommended.

Dose Forms Available
- Capsules: 25 mg, 50 mg, 75 mg

Pharmacokinetics of Clomipramine

Clomipramine has a long half-life. The mean half-life of a single 150-mg dose is 32 hours, and the mean half-life of its major metabolite, desmethylclomipramine, is 69 hours. Steady-state serum levels usually occur within 1 to 2 weeks at a given daily dosage. Children and adolescents under 15 years of age had significantly lower plasma concentrations for a given dose than did adults (package insert). Dugas et al. (1980) reported that peak plasma clomipramine levels were achieved 3 to 4 hours after ingestion in the three children they studied and reported an apparent plasma terminal half-life of 11.9 to 17.3 hours. The bioavailability of clomipramine is not significantly affected by being taken with food, and administering it during initial titration in divided doses with meals helps to reduce gastrointestinal side effects. Clomipramine is metabolized in large part to its major bioactive metabolite desmethylclomipramine; both compounds are ultimately metabolized into their glucuronide conjugates by the liver. The metabolites are excreted through the bile duct and the kidneys.

Untoward Effects of Clomipramine

The most significant risk of clomipramine appears to be the development of seizures. Risk for seizures is cumulative and increased from 0.64% at 90 days to 1.45% at 1 year. Other untoward effects that occur in children and adolescents include somnolence, tremor, dizziness, headache, sleep disorders, increased sweating, gastrointestinal effects (dry mouth, constipation, and dyspepsia), anorexia, fatigue, cardiovascular effects (postural hypotension, palpitations, tachycardia, and syncope), abnormalities of vision, urinary retention, and dysmenorrhea in females and ejaculation failure in males (package insert). Because of reports of blood dyscrasias, a complete blood count should be determined in patients who develop fever and sore throat during the course of treatment.

Dugas and his colleagues (1980) reported in their study of 8 children and 28 adolescents administered clomipramine for enuresis or depressive symptomatology that the incidence of untoward effects was clearly related to the clomipramine plasma concentration. Untoward effects occurred in about 15% to 20% of patients with plasma clomipramine levels below 60 ng/ml and were present in over 90% of cases with serum levels above 90 ng/ml. Hypotension occurred only in cases with serum levels above 80 ng/ml. No discernible relationship was found between untoward effects and plasma levels of desmethylclomipramine.

Investigational Reports of Interest

Clomipramine in the Treatment of Obsessive-Compulsive Disorder in Children and Adolescents

There are few published studies on the use of clomipramine in children and adolescents diagnosed with obsessive-compulsive disorder. Those of Flament et al. (1985, 1987) and of Leonard et al. (1989) include some children below the age of 10 years and are summarized briefly below.

Clomipramine was found to be significantly superior to placebo in a placebo-controlled double-blind cross-over study of 19 subjects whose ages ranged from 10 to 18 years (mean, 14.5 ± 2.3 years) who were diagnosed with severe primary obsessive-compulsive disorder (Flament et al., 1985). The dose range was 100 to 200 mg/day (mean, 141 ± 30 mg/day). The experimental data suggested that clomipramine has a direct antiobsessional action that is independent of any antidepressant effect. In fact, 10 of the subjects had been previously treated with other tricyclics without significant benefit. Flament et al. (1987) increased the number of their subjects to 29 (mean age, 13.9 ± 2.5 years; range, 8 to 18 years) and reported the continued efficacy of clomipramine; the mean daily dose of clomipramine was 134 ± 33 mg/day.

Leonard et al. (1989) compared the efficacy of clomipramine and desipramine in the treatment of severe primary obsessive-compulsive disorder in 49 child and adolescent subjects (31 males and 18 females) (mean age, 13.86 ± 2.87 years; range, 7 to 19 years). In a 10-week cross-over design, clomipramine was markedly superior to desipramine in decreasing obsessive-compulsive symptoms on several rating scales. In addition, when desipramine was administered following improvement on clomipramine, subjects experienced relapse rates similar to those for placebo in the Flament (1985) study.

Administration of clomipramine was begun at 25 mg/day for children weighing 25 kg or less and at 50 mg/day for subjects weighing over 25 kg (Leonard et al., 1989). Dosage was increased weekly by an amount equal to each subject's initial dose. Maximum dosage did not exceed 250 mg/day or 5 mg/kg/day. The mean dose of clomipramine at week 5 was 150 ± 53 mg/day, with a range of 50 to 250 mg/day. The most common side effects reported were dry mouth, tremor, tiredness, dizziness, difficulty sleeping, sweating, constipation, poor appetite, and weakness.

Evidence at the present time suggests that clomipramine is the drug of choice for children and adolescents with severe obsessive-compulsive disorder, although it has not been approved by the FDA for advertising as effective and safe in treating children under 10 years of age.

Clomipramine in the Treatment of Attention Deficit Hyperactivity Disorder

Garfinkel and colleagues (1983) compared the clinical efficacy of methylphenidate, desipramine, and clomipramine in a double-blind placebo-controlled cross-over study of 12 males (mean age, 7.3 years; range, 5.9 to 11.6 years) diagnosed with attention deficit disorder who required day hospital or inpatient treatment for severe impulsiveness, attention deficit, and aggression. The mean dose of clomipramine was 85 mg/day and did not exceed 100 mg or 3.5 mg/kg/day for any subject. Methylphenidate was significantly better than the other three conditions in improving overall classroom functioning as rated on the Conners Scale by teachers ($P < .005$) and program child care workers ($P < .001$). Clomipramine, however, was significantly better than desipramine in reducing scores reflecting aggressivity, impulsivity, and depressive/affective symptoms. Based on these data, clomipramine would merit further study in treating children and adolescents with ADHD who do not respond satisfactorily to stimulant medication.

Clomipramine in the Treatment of Enuresis

Dugas et al. (1980) administered clomipramine to 10 enuretic children. A therapeutic effect was observed at plasma clomipramine concentrations of 20 to 60 ng/ml, while lower and higher levels were associated with lack of therapeutic efficacy or untoward effects. In a later report the sample was increased to 31 enuretic children (Morselli et al., 1983). Of the 21 who had good therapeutic outcomes, 16 (76%) had plasma steady-state clomipramine concentrations greater than 15 ng/ml, whereas only 3 of the 10 nonresponders has plasma levels this high. The plasma level differences between the responders and the nonresponders was significant ($P < .05$).

Clomipramine in the Treatment of Depressive Symptoms

Dugas et al. (1980) treated 1 boy, 8.5 years old, and 25 adolescents, 13 to 19 years old, who had significant depressive symptomatology with clomipramine. Clomipramine doses ranged from 0.24 to 2.93 mg/kg/day. Sixteen cases received other psychoactive medication simultaneously. Twelve of the 26 patients responded positively. Final diagnoses of these patients were school phobia (3), anorexia nervosa (6), manic-depressive psychosis (1), depression (5), and depressive reactions in behavior disorders or borderline personalities (11). Two patients had no therapeutic response, 1 had a minimal response, 11 had moderate improvement, 3 had "good" results, and 9 had excellent results. The patients diagnosed with anorexia responded least favorably; only 2 had a good response, while 4 of the 5 diagnosed with depression had excellent responses. Similar plasma levels of clomipramine were present in both responders and nonresponders; however, nonresponders had proportionally higher levels of desmethylclomipramine.

Clomipramine in the Treatment of School Phobia (Separation Anxiety)

Berney et al. (1981) treated 52 children diagnosed with school refusal, which consisted of a neurotic disorder with a marked reluctance to attend school for at least 4 weeks' duration and was frequently associated with depressive features. The study was double-blind and placebo controlled and lasted for 12 weeks. Forty-six patients aged 9 to 14 years old completed the study; 19 were on placebo, and 27 were on clomipramine. Clomipramine total daily dosage was titrated slowly to 40 mg/day for 9- and 10-year-olds; 50 mg/day for 11- and 12-year-olds; and 75 mg/day for 13- and 14-year-olds. There was no evidence that clomipramine was superior to placebo in reducing separation anxiety and neurotic behavior or being specific for depression. The authors, however, noted they used proportionally lower doses of clomipramine than the doses of imipramine used in studies reporting its efficacy in treating school phobia/separation anxiety.

MONOAMINE OXIDASE INHIBITORS

There are two forms monoamine oxidase (MAO), which are distinguished by their substrate specificity. Type A MAO deaminates or deactivates norepinephrine, serotonin, and normetanephrine; and Type B MAO deaminates dopamine and phenylethylamine (Zametkin & Rapoport, 1987).

Monoamine oxidase inhibitors (MAOIs) are primarily used in treating adults with depressive disorders that are unresponsive to antidepressants of other classes. MAOIs presently FDA-approved and marketed in the United States include isocarboxazid (Marplan), phenelzine sulfate (Nardil), and tranylcypromine sulfate (Parnate). The first two drugs have been approved for use only in individuals at least 16 years of age, and the latter drug only for adults.

MAOIs that have been used in children and adolescents include clorgyline (a selective MAO-A inhibitor), tranylcypromine sulfate (Parnate) (a mixed MAO-A and MAO-B inhibitor), phenelzine sulfate (Nardil), and L-deprenyl (a selective central MAO-B inhibitor). Because of the potentially very serious drug interactions and untoward effects of MAOIs, their use in children and adolescents is not usually recommended, and only a few research reports in this age group will be reviewed.

Special Considerations in Using MAOIs

It is critical to have a minimum of a 2-week washout period after stopping an MAOI and beginning a tricyclic or when changing from one MAOI to another MAOI. It is also contraindicated to add a tricyclic antidepressant when an MAOI is already being used, although the reverse has been done; that is, an MAOI can be added to an ongoing treatment regimen to augment a tricyclic that has been only partially effective (Ryan et al., 1988b). If patients are on MAOIs and will be in areas that are not rapidly accessible to medical treatment, they may be given several 25-mg chlorpromazine tablets to take should they accidentally ingest tyramine and become symptomatic (Ryan et al., 1988b). Pare et al. (1982) suggested that a combination of tricyclics and MAOIs might provide a relative protection against tyramine-induced hypertension, or "cheese effect," which may occur with dietary indiscretions while taking MAOIs; however, this is not common practice at the present time.

Contraindications for MAOI Administration

Known hypersensitivity to an MAOI, pheochromocytoma, congestive heart failure, liver disease or abnormal liver function are contraindications.

MAOIs must not be prescribed if a tricyclic antidepressant, (however, see Ryan et al., 1988b, for a different opinion), another MAOI, or buspirone hydrochloride has been taken within the preceding 2 weeks.

Other contraindications usually found more frequently in older patients also exist. In addition, the patient must not be unreliable or be unable to keep to a strict diet avoiding foods with high tyramine or dopamine concentrations.

Interactions of MAOIs with Other Drugs

Ingestion of tyramine can cause a hypertensive crisis. Hence foods rich in tyramine, such as cheese, wine, beer, yeast derivatives, some beans, and others, must be avoided.

Concomitant use with tricyclic antidepressants should be avoided as hypertensive crises or severe seizures have been reported with such combinations (See Ryan et al., for a different opinion).

Use with sympathomimetic drugs such as amphetamines,

methylphenidate, cocaine, dopamine, caffeine, epinephrine, nor-epinephrine, and related compounds may cause a hypertensive crisis.

Other drug interactions occur as well.

Untoward Effects of MAOIs

MAOIs may cause significant orthostatic hypotension, dizziness, headache, sleep disturbances, sedation, fatigue, weakness, hyperreflexia, dry mouth, and gastrointestinal disturbances; other untoward effects occur as well.

Investigational Reports of Interest

MAOIs in the Treatment of Adolescent Depression

Ryan and his colleagues reported an open clinical trial of tranylcypromine sulfate and phenelzine sulfate, both alone and in combination with a tricyclic antidepressant, in which 23 adolescents diagnosed with major depressive disorder who had responded inadequately to tricyclic antidepressants were treated with these MAOIs (Ryan et al., 1988b). Seventy-four percent (17) had a fair to good antidepressant response; however, because of dietary noncompliance the MAOI was discontinued in 4 subjects and only 57% (13) of the subjects continued on the medication. The authors concluded that MAOIs appeared to be useful in treating some adolescents with major depression that has not responded satisfactorily to tricyclic antidepressants. During the study a total of 7 (30%) had purposeful or accidental dietary noncompliance, and the authors emphasized that only very reliable adolescents are suitable for treatment with MAOIs (Ryan et al., 1988b).

MAOIs in the Treatment of ADHD

Zametkin et al. (1985) conducted a double-blind cross-over study of 14 boys (mean age, 9.2 ± 1.5 years) who were diagnosed with attention deficit disorder with hyperactivity. The authors compared dextroamphetamine with either clorgyline, a selective MAO-A inhibitor (6 subjects), or tranylcypromine sulfate, a mixed MAO-A and MAO-B inhibitor) (8 subjects). Both MAOIs had immediate, clinically significant effects (in contrast to delayed effects when used as an antidepressant), which were clinically indistinguishable from those of dextroamphetamine.

Zametkin and Rapoport (1987) reported that M. Donnelly had administered 15 mg/day of L-deprenyl, a selective MAO-B inhibitor, to 14 hyperactive children with relatively little therapeutic effect. The authors suggested that the fact that a type A MAOI and a mixed MAOI showed therapeutic efficacy in children with ADHD but a type B MAOI did not supported the hypothesis that dysregulation of the noradrenergic system is important in the etiology of ADHD (Zametkin and Rapoport, 1987).

At the present time, the use of MAOIs in the treatment of ADHD must be regarded as investigational and cannot be recommended.

Fluoxetine Hydrochloride (Prozac)

Fluoxetine hydrochloride, recently approved for the treatment of depression in adults, is chemically unrelated to tricyclic, tetracyclic, and other currently approved antidepressants. Safety and effectiveness in children have not been established.

Fluoxetine's antidepressant effect is thought to be related to its specific and selective inhibition of serotonin reuptake by CNS neurons. Its specific action on the serotonergic system appears to take place at the serotonin reuptake pump, not at a neurotransmitter receptor site, and fluoxetine appears to have no significant pharmacological effect on norepinephrine or dopamine uptake (Bergstrom et al., 1988).

Indications for Use in Child and Adolescent Psychiatry
　　Fluoxetine is only approved for use in older adolescents and adults for the treatment of depression.

Dosage Schedule for Children and Adolescents
- Children and younger adolescents: Not approved. At the present time, the safety and efficacy of fluoxetine for children and younger adolescents remains to be elucidated, and its use in this population should be regarded as investigational.
- Older adolescents (at least 18 years old, i.e., adult dosage): An initial morning dose of 20 mg/day is recommended; there is evidence that this may frequently be the optimal dose (Altamura et al., 1988). If significant untoward affects develop, the dose may be lowered to 20 mg every other day. The full antidepressant action may take 4 weeks or longer to develop. If adequate clinical response does not occur after several weeks, the dosage may be increased gradually to a maximum of 80 mg/day. It is recommended that once 20 mg/day is exceeded, the medication be taken in divided portions twice daily, in the morning and at noon. Food does not seem to affect significantly the bioavailability of fluoxetine.

Dose Forms Available
- Pulvules: 20 mg

Pharmacokinetics of Fluoxetine

Peak plasma levels of fluoxetine at usual clinical doses occur after 6 to 8 hours. Fluoxetine is metabolized by the liver; active and inactive metabolites are excreted by the kidneys. About 95% of fluoxetine is bound to plasma proteins. The elimination half-life is 2 to 3 days for fluoxetine and 7 to 9 days for norfluoxetine, its active metabolite. It may take up to several weeks for steady-state plasma levels to be achieved, but once obtained they remain steady (Bergstrom et al., 1988; package insert).

Contraindications for Fluoxetine Administration

Known hypersensitivity to the drug is an absolute contraindication.

Fluoxetine should not be administered to any patient who has received an MAOI within 5 weeks (35 days).

The drug should be administered with caution if impaired liver function is present.

Interactions of Fluoxetine with Other Drugs

The use of fluoxetine with other psychoactive drugs has not been systematically studied as yet.

Severe reactions may occur if an MAOI and fluoxetine are administered simultaneously or sufficient time has not elapsed after stopping either of these drugs before beginning the other.

When used with tricyclic antidepressants, their plasma levels may be significantly increased.

Agitation, restlessness, and gastrointestinal symptoms have occurred when used concurrently with tryptophan.

Diazepam clearance was significantly prolonged in some patients administered both drugs.

Untoward Effects of Fluoxetine

Wernicke (1985) and Cooper (1988) have reviewed the safety and untoward effects of fluoxetine. The most frequent troublesome untoward effects are nausea, weight loss, anxiety, nervousness, insomnia, and excessive sweating. They are reported more frequently, and anticholinergic effects and sedation less frequently, than with the tricyclics.

Several studies, including some that were placebo controlled, have found fluoxetine's therapeutic efficacy to be comparable to that of the tricyclics (imipramine, amitriptyline, and doxepine) in treating adults with major depressive disorder (for reviews see

Benfield et al., 1986; Lader, 1988). There is also some evidence fluoxetine may be helpful in treating obsessive-compulsive disorder (Benfield et al., 1986).

Investigational Reports of Interest

Fluoxetine in the Treatment of Child and Adolescent Major Depressive Disorder

Joshi and colleagues (1989) reported on their treatment with fluoxetine of 14 patients (8 males, 6 females) ranging in age from 9 to 15 years (average age, 11.25 years) who were diagnosed with major depression by DSM-III-R (APA, 1987) criteria and who had not responded adequately to tricyclic antidepressants, had serious untoward effects from tricyclics, or could not be treated with tricyclics for medical reasons. Ten (71.4%) of the subjects responded favorably within 6 weeks to fluoxetine 20 mg administered in the morning. Side effects were limited to transient nausea and hyperactivity in one patient each and did not require discontinuation of the drug.

Fluoxetine in the Treatment of Children and Adolescents with Obsessive-Compulsive Disorder or Obsessive-Compulsive Disorder and Tourette's Disorder

In an open clinical study, Riddle et al. (1990) treated with fluoxetine 10 children (5 males, 5 females) ranging in age from 8 to 15 years (average age, 12.2 years) diagnosed with obsessive-compulsive disorder only or with both obsessive-compulsive disorder and Tourette's disorder. Dosage ranged from 10 to 40 mg/day, with 80% of the patients receiving 20 mg/day; duration of treatment ranged from 4 to 20 weeks. Four of the patients with Tourette's disorder received concomitantly additional medication for treatment of their tics. Fifty percent were considered responders to fluoxetine and were rated much improved; response rates were similar in patients with obsessive-compulsive disorder alone and in those with both diagnoses. The most common untoward effect was behavioral agitation/activation, characterized by increased motor activity and pressured speech. It occurred in 40% of the patients and usually started within the first few days; symptoms were most severe during the 1st 2 to 3 weeks but remained until medication was discontinued. No significant changes in blood pressure, pulse, weight, laboratory tests, or ECG were observed (Riddle et al., 1990).

BUPROPION HYDROCHLORIDE (WELLBUTRIN)

Bupropion hydrochloride is an antidepressant of the aminoketone class. It is not related chemically to the tricyclics, tetracyclics, or other known antidepressants. It has been approved by the FDA for treating depression in individuals at least 18 years of age.

Indications in Child and Adolescent Psychiatry
- Children and adolescents under age 18: Not approved for any use.
- Adolescents at least 18 years of age: Used to treat depression, especially major depressive disorder.

Dosage Schedule for Children and Adolescents
- Children and adolescents under 18 years of age: Not recommended.
- Adolescents at least 18 years of age: An initial dosage of 100 mg twice daily is suggested. Based on clinical response, this may be increased to 100 mg three times daily, but not before day 4 of treatment. If no clinical improvement occurs within 4 weeks, dosage may gradually be increased. Because of increased risk of seizure, a dose of 150 mg should not be exceeded within a 4-hour time period. The maximum daily dosage should not exceed 450 mg.

Dose Forms Available
- Tablets: 75 mg, 100 mg

Contraindications for Bupropion Hydrochloride Administration

Known hypersensitivity to bupropion hydrochloride and seizure disorders are absolute contraindications.

A current or prior diagnosis of bulimia or anorexia nervosa is also a contraindication, as a higher incidence of seizures is reported when bupropion is administered to such patients.

This drug should not be administered concurrently with an MAOI. At least a 14-day period off MAOIs should precede initiation of treatment with bupropion hydrochloride.

Concurrent administration with any drug that reduces the seizure threshold is a relative contraindication.

Interactions of Bupropion Hydrochloride with Other Drugs

There are relatively few data available on this subject. Increased adverse experiences were reported when the drug was administered concomitantly with L-dopa. MAOIs may increase the acute toxicity of bupropion.

Untoward Effects of Bupropion Hydrochloride

Of particular clinical concern is the finding that seizures have been associated with about 4 of 1000 (0.4%) patients treated with bupropion at doses of 450 mg/day or less. This is about fourfold the incidence of seizures reported with other approved antidepressants, and the incidence of seizures increases with higher daily doses. On the other hand, Clay et al. (1988) note that bupropion's positive effects on memory performance may be unique among antidepressants, and that other antidepressants either have no effect or a negative effect on memory performance.

The most common untoward effects were reported to be agitation, dry mouth, insomnia, headache, nausea, vomiting, constipation, and tremor.

Ferguson and Simeon (1984) reported no adverse (or positive) effects on cognition on a cognitive battery in 17 children with attention deficit disorder or conduct disorders who were treated in an open trial with bupropion.

Investigational Reports of Interest

Bupropion Hydrochloride in the Treatment of ADHD

Clay et al. (1988) reported that bupropion hydrochloride was safe and efficacious in treating prepubertal children diagnosed with attention deficit hyperactivity disorder (ADHD). The authors' clinical impression was that children with additional prominent symptoms of conduct disorder responded particularly well to bupropion.

Thirty prepubertal children diagnosed with ADHD were enrolled in a double-blind placebo-controlled study and individually titrated to optimal doses of bupropion (Clay et al., 1988). Optimal doses ranged from 100 to 250 mg/day (3.1 to 7.1 mg/kg/day; mean, 5.3 ± 1 mg/kg/day). Subjects receiving bupropion showed statistically significant improvement on the Clinical Global Impressions Improvement and Severity Rating scales, the Self-Rating Scale, and on digit symbol and delayed recall on the Selective Reminding Test. Improvement that did not reach significance was also reported on the Conners Parent Questionnaire and the Conners Teacher Questionnaire. The only serious side effect noted was an allergic rash in two children.

Clay et al. (1988) also noted that some children who had previously not responded satisfactorily to stimulants had a good response to bupropion. On the other hand, some subjects who had never received stimulants and who did not respond well to bupropion responded well when methylphenidate was openly prescribed at a later time.

Casat et al. (1989) administered bupropion to 20 children and placebo to 10 children in a parallel groups design, double-blind comparison study. All subjects were diagnosed with attention deficit disorder with hyperactivity. Decreases in symptom severity and overall clinical improvement were noted in physician ratings, and hyperactivity in the classroom settings was significantly decreased on the Conners Teachers Questionnaire.

Although confirmation of these findings is needed, bupropion may be an alternative treatment for ADHD that does not respond to standard therapies.

6

Lithium Carbonate

INTRODUCTION

At the present time, lithium carbonate is approved by the FDA only for the treatment of manic episodes of bipolar disorders and for maintenance therapy of bipolar patients with a history of mania in persons at least 12 years of age. Over the past 2 decades, however, lithium carbonate has been investigated in the treatment of many child and adolescent disorders, but especially in the treatment of children with severe aggression directed toward self or others, children with bipolar or similar disorders, and behaviorally disturbed children whose parents are known lithium responders. One major impetus for this research is that antipsychotics, which are frequently used to control severe behavioral disorders and sometimes mania, may cause cognitive dulling when used in sufficient dosage to control symptoms and carry significant risk of causing tardive dyskinesia when used on a long-term basis (Platt et al., 1984).

PHARMACOKINETICS OF LITHIUM CARBONATE

The lithium ion is readily absorbed from the gastrointestinal tract and is most commonly administered in the form of lithium carbonate (Li_2CO_3), a highly soluble salt. Peak plasma concentrations occur within 2 to 4 hours, and complete absorption takes place within about 8 hours (Baldessarini, 1990). About 95% of a single dose of lithium is excreted by the kidneys with up to two-thirds of an acute dose being excreted within 6 to 12 hours. The serum half-life is approximately 20 to 24 hours. Depletion of the sodium ion causes a clinically significant degree of lithium retention by the kidneys. Steady-state serum lithium levels typically occur within 5 to 8 days following repeated identical daily doses of lithium carbonate. Although lithium pharmacokinetics differ considerably among individuals, they are fairly stable over time for a given person (Baldessarini & Stephens, 1970).

Vitiello et al. (1988) studied the pharmacokinetics of lithium carbonate in 9 children aged 9 years to 12 years. The children had a trend toward a shorter elimination half-life of lithium and a significantly higher total renal clearance of lithium. The clinical significance of this is that a steady state of lithium serum levels is reached more rapidly in children than in adults, and therapeutic levels can be achieved more quickly.

CONTRAINDICATIONS FOR LITHIUM CARBONATE ADMINISTRATION

Administration of lithium carbonate is relatively contraindicated in individuals with significant renal or cardiovascular disease, severe debilitation, severe dehydration, or sodium depletion, as these conditions are associated with a very high risk of lithium toxicity. Patients with such disorders should be thoroughly assessed, usually with consultation with the person providing medical care, prior to beginning lithium therapy.

Adolescents who may purposely or accidentally become pregnant should not be administered lithium, particularly in early pregnancy, except under urgent circumstances. Lithium carbonate is associated with a significant increase in cardiac teratogenicity, and especially with Ebstein's anomaly. A significantly increased incidence of other cardiac anomalies has also been reported. Källén and Tandberg (1983) reported that 7% of the infants of women who used lithium in early pregnancy had serious heart defects other than Ebstein's anomaly.

Significant thyroid disease is a relative contraindication to lithium carbonate therapy; however, with careful monitoring of thyroid function and the use of supplemental thyroid preparations when necessary, it may be used when other drugs are not effective and the potential benefits outweigh the risks.

INTERACTIONS OF LITHIUM CARBONATE WITH OTHER DRUGS

There are several reports that increased neuroleptic toxicity with an encephalopathic syndrome or neuroleptic malignant syndrome may occur when lithium and neuroleptics are used concomitantly, but this has usually been seen with high doses. The simultaneous use of lithium and neuroleptics, however, may be indicated in some cases of mania or schizoaffective psychoses, and many patients have received both a neuroleptic and lithium with no untoward effects.

Lithium serum concentration and increased risk of neurotoxic lithium effects may occur when carbamazepine and lithium are used simultaneously, as carbamazepine decreases lithium renal clearance.

Many other drugs may potentially increase or decrease serum lithium levels by influencing its absorption or excretion by the kidneys; for example, tetracyclines increase lithium levels.

LITHIUM TOXICITY

One major difficulty associated with the administration of lithium carbonate is its low therapeutic index; lithium toxicity is closely related to serum levels and may occur at doses close to therapeutic levels. Untoward or side effects are those unwanted symptoms that occur at therapeutic serum lithium levels, while toxic effects occur when serum lithium levels exceed therapeutic levels.

Lithium toxicity may be heralded by diarrhea, vomiting, mild ataxia, coarse tremor, muscular weakness and fasciculation, drowsiness, sedation, slurred speech, and impaired coordination. Patients and/or their caretakers must be made familiar with the symptoms of early lithium toxicity and instructed to discontinue lithium immediately and contact their physician if such signs occur. Increasingly severe and life-threatening toxic effects, including cardiac arrhythmias and severe central nervous system difficulties such as impaired consciousness, confusion, stupor, seizures, coma, and death may occur with further elevations in serum lithium levels.

No specific treatment for lithium toxicity is available. If signs of early lithium toxicity appear, the drug should be withheld, lithium levels determined, and the medication resumed at a lower dosage only after 24 to 48 hours. Severe lithium toxicity is life threatening and requires hospital admission, treatments to reduce the concentration of the lithium ion, and supportive measures.

Lithium's low therapeutic index and its pharmacokinetics make it necessary to administer lithium carbonate tablets or immediate release capsules in divided doses, usually three or four times daily, to maintain therapeutic serum levels without toxicity. Even controlled release tablets must be administered every 12 hours. It is essential that a laboratory capable of determining serum lithium levels rapidly and accurately be readily available to the clinician. For accuracy and serial comparisons, determinations of serum lithium levels should be made when lithium concentrations are relatively stable, and at the same time each day. Typically, blood is drawn 12 hours after the last dose of lithium and immediately before the morning dose.

Lithium saliva levels have also been used to monitor lithium levels in children, which avoids the necessity of repeated venipunctures, an upsetting experience for some children and adolescents. Perry et al. (1984) reported that saliva lithium levels in 15 children diagnosed with undersocialized aggressive conduct disorder averaged about 2.5 times higher than serum lithium levels, with saliva/serum ratios for individual children ranging from 1.56 to 3.99. Weller et al. (1987) found that saliva lithium levels were about 1.82 times serum levels in 14 prepubertal children receiving lithium for treatment of bipolar disorder. Saliva/serum lithium ratios in these children ranged from 1.50 to 2.32. Vitiello et al. (1988) reported saliva lithium levels to be 2.84 times those of serum lithium levels in 9 children, 6 of whom were diagnosed with conduct disorder and 3 of whom were diagnosed with adjustment disorders. Saliva/serum lithium ratios in these children ranged from 2.08 to 3.88. Bernstein (1988) found that in adults the ratio of saliva lithium levels to serum lithium levels varied from 1:1 to as high as 3:1. Despite the rather marked interindividual variability in the saliva/serum ratio, it appears to be relatively constant for a given individual. Therefore, to be clinically useful, a stable saliva/serum lithium level must be calculated for each patient.

Although some patients who are unusually sensitive to lithium may exhibit toxic effects at serum levels below 1 mEq/liter, for most patients mild to moderate untoward effects occur at serum levels between 1.5 and 2 mEq/liter, and moderate to severe reactions occur at levels of 2 mEq/liter and above. Younger subjects may be at greater risk than adults for developing untoward effects at lower serum lithium levels. Many untoward effects have been reported to occur in children at serum levels well below 1 mEq/liter (Campbell et al., 1984a). The most common side effects of lithium carbonate in 36 children aged 3 years to 13 years and diagnosed with conduct disorder (N = 24), infantile autism (N = 8), or other (N = 4) were weight gain in 44.4%, excessive sedation in 27.8%, decreased motor activity in 25%, and stomachache, vomiting, tremor, and/or irritability in 19.4% of patients (Campbell et al., 1984a).

Lithium decreases sodium reuptake by the renal tubules; hence adequate sodium intake must be maintained. This is especially important if there is significant sodium loss during illness (e.g., sweating, vomiting, or diarrhea) or because of changes in diet or elimination of electrolytes. The importance of adequate ingestion of ordinary table salt and fluids should be emphasized. Caution during hot weather or vigorous exertion has been advised, as additional salt loss and concomitant dehydration secondary to pronounced diaphoresis may cause the serum lithium levels of patients on maintenance lithium to increase and move into the toxic range. This may also be true of sweating caused by elevated body temperature secondary to infection or heat without exercise (e.g., sauna), but some evidence suggests that heavy sweating caused by exercise may result in lowered rather than elevated serum lithium levels. Jefferson et al. (1982) studied four healthy athletes who were stabilized on lithium for a week prior to running a 20-km race. At the end of the race, the subjects were dehydrated, but their serum lithium levels had decreased by 20%. The authors found that the sweat-to-serum ratio for the lithium ion was about four times greater than that for the sodium ion. These authors concluded that strenuous exercise with extensive perspiration was more likely to decrease rather than increase serum lithium levels, and patients were more likely to require either no change or an increase in dosage of lithium to maintain therapeutic levels than a decrease in dosage. The authors do caution, however, that any conditions that significantly alter fluid and electrolyte balance, including strenuous exercise with heavy sweating, should be carefully monitored with serum lithium levels.

UNTOWARD EFFECTS OF LITHIUM CARBONATE

Lithium carbonate is frequently reported to have untoward effects early in the course of treatment. Most of these diminish or disappear during the 1st weeks of treatment.

These early untoward effects include fine tremor (unresponsive to antiparkinsonism drugs), polydipsia, and polyuria that may occur during initial treatment and persist or be variably present throughout treatment. Nausea and malaise or general discomfort may initially occur but usually subside with ongoing treatment. Weight gain, headache, and other gastrointestinal complaints such as diarrhea may also occur. Taking the lithium with meals or after meals or increasing the dosage more gradually may be helpful in controlling gastrointestinal symptoms.

Later untoward effects are often related to serum level, including levels in the therapeutic range, and include continued hand tremor that may worsen, polydipsia, polyuria, weight gain and edema, thyroid and renal abnormalities, dermatological abnormalities, fatigue, leukocytosis, and other symptoms. As serum levels increase, toxicity increases and other, more severe untoward effects discussed above under toxicity appear.

Abnormalities in renal functioning (diminution of renal concentrating ability) and morphological structure (glomerular and interstitial fibrosis and nephron atrophy) have been reported in adults on long-term lithium maintenance. Occasional proteinuria was reported in a 14-year-old girl (Lena et al., 1978). Vetro et al. (1985) reported that after 1 year of lithium treatment, one child developed polyuria with daytime enuresis and impaired renal concentration. Other parameters of renal function did not change, and polyuria ceased within a few days after lithium was discontinued. Five other children on long-term lithium therapy showed transient albuminuria that remitted spontaneously, and discontinuation of treatment was not necessary (Vetro et al., 1985).

Lithium also may interfere with thyroid function, with decreased circulating hormones and increased TSH. Vetro et al. (1985) reported that two children developed goiter with normal function after 1.5 to 2 years of lithium therapy.

Neuroleptic malignant syndrome has been reported in patients who were administered neuroleptics and lithium simultaneously.

Dostal (1972) reported specific untoward effects of lithium in 14 retarded adolescent males that interfered with patient management, despite significant therapeutic gains. Polydipsia, polyuria, and nocturnal enuresis were so severe as to alienate staff who cared for the youngsters. These symptoms remitted within 2 weeks after discontinuing lithium (Dostal, 1972).

PREMEDICATION WORK-UP AND PERIODIC MONITORING FOR LITHIUM TREATMENT

Routine Laboratory Tests

Complete Blood Count with Differential

Lithium frequently causes a clinically insignificant and reversible elevation of white blood cells, with counts commonly between 10,000 and 15,000 cells/mm^3. The lithium-induced leukocytosis characteristically shows neutrophilia (increased polymorphonuclear leukocytes) and lymphocytopenia (Reisberg & Gershon, 1979). This leukocytosis can usually be differentiated from one caused by infection, as the increase in neutrophils is in more mature forms, whereas in infection younger forms predominate. Lithium may also increase platelet counts.

Serum Electrolytes

Serum electrolyte levels should be determined in particular to verify that sodium ion levels are normal, as hyponatremia decreases lithium excretion by the renal tubules.

Pregnancy Test

Lithium crosses the placenta, and data from birth registries suggest teratogenicity with increased abnormalities, including cardiac malformations, especially Ebstein's anomaly. Lithium is relatively contraindicated during pregnancy but especially during the first trimester. Infants born to mothers taking lithium appear to be at increased risk for hypotonia, lethargy, cyanosis, and ECG changes (United States Pharmacopeial Dispensing Information [USPDI], 1990). All females who could be pregnant should be tested prior to initiation of lithium therapy and warned that because of its teratogenic potential for the fetus, they should take care not to become pregnant while taking lithium.

Renal Function Tests

Baseline assessment of renal functioning is essential, as this is the primary route of elimination of lithium. For healthy children and adolescents, a baseline serum creatinine and urinalysis are usually adequate (Jefferson et al., 1987). If kidney disease is suspected or abnormalities found, a more thorough evaluation including tests such as urinalysis (including specific gravity), blood urea nitrogen (BUN) level, 24-hour urine volume, and 24-

hour urine for creatinine clearance and protein should be performed and the patient referred to a renal consultant if necessary.

Thyroid Function Tests

Lithium causes thyroid abnormalities primarily by decreasing the release of thyroid hormones. This causes such findings as euthyroid goiter; hypothyroidism; decreased triiodothyronine (T_3), thyroxine (T_4), and protein-bound iodine (PBI) levels; and elevated I^{131} and thyroid-stimulating hormone (TSH) levels in between 5% and 15% of patients receiving long-term lithium therapy (Jefferson et al., 1987). Hypothyroidism resulting from lithium treatment is thought to be related to preexisting Hashimoto's thyroiditis, suggesting that determining antithyroid antibodies as part of the work-up may be useful (Rosse et al., 1989). Recommended baseline studies include triiodothyronine resin uptake (T_3RU), and TSH levels.

Cardiovascular Function Tests

Various cardiac conduction and repolarization abnormalities (e.g., bradycardia), and reversible ECG abnormalities have been reported in a significant percentage of adults receiving lithium. ECG changes commonly include benign, reversible T wave changes (flattening, isoelectricity, and inversion of T waves), which are dose dependent, and an increase in the P-Q interval (Jefferson et al., 1987). It has been hypothesized that lithium's cardiotoxic effects result from its displacing and substituting for intracellular potassium. A baseline ECG should be obtained routinely in patients over age 40 or those who have any history or clinical suggestions of cardiovascular disease. Although not considered mandatory in young, healthy patients, a baseline ECG is justifiable and useful to have for comparison should cardiovascular abnormalities develop at some later time. If patients have or develop cardiac abnormalities, frequent ECG monitoring should be done and the advice of a cardiac consultant sought. In other patients it is prudent to repeat the ECG at the time of scheduled routine physical examinations.

Calcium Metabolism Tests

Lithium may increase renal calcium reabsorption, resulting in hypocalciuria (Jefferson et al., 1987). Lithium may also cause hyperparathyroidism with hypercalcemia and hypophosphatemia, with resulting decreased bone formation or density in children. If abnormal results occur, parathyroid hormone (parathormone) levels may be determined. Lithium may also replace calcium in bone formation, especially in immature bones (USPDI, 1990). A baseline calcium level should be determined in children and adolescents, but a baseline parathormone level is not usually recommended.

Electroencephalogram

Bennett el al. (1983) reported that optimal doses of lithium caused worsening of conduct-disordered children's EEGs in statistically significant numbers. Paroxysmal and focal EEG abnormalities in particular were increased over pretreatment EEGs. EEG worsening, however, did not correlate with clinical symptoms of toxicity, and children receiving lithium showed significantly more behavioral improvement than those receiving placebo.

Although an EEG is not required as a baseline work-up for normal healthy youngsters, if EEG abnormalities or a seizure disorder is known to exist, a baseline EEG should be obtained and the EEG periodically monitored. Lithium levels should be determined the morning that the EEG is performed, to facilitate correlation of EEG changes and serum lithium levels.

Periodic Monitoring

As there is little information on the long-term effects of lithium on the development and maturation of children and adolescents, periodic monitoring of thyroid, kidney, and cardiac functioning is particularly important. It is recommended that TSH, BUN, and serum creatinine levels be determined at approximately 6-month intervals. When there is a concern about renal function, 24-hour urine volume, creatinine clearance, and protein excretion should also be determined. If a suggestion of thyroid abnormality arises, T_3 and T_4 levels should also be determined (Rosse et al., 1989).

Lithium Carbonate (Eskalith, Lithane, Lithobid), Lithium Citrate Syrup (Cibalith-S)

Indications in Child and Adolescent Psychiatry
FDA approved for the treatment of manic episodes of manic-depressive illness and maintenance therapy of manic-depressive patients with a history of mania who are at least 12 years of age. Significant

normalization of manic symptomatology may require up to 3 weeks of lithium carbonate therapy; hence concomitant use of antipsychotic medication may be initially required for more rapid control of manic symptoms.

Dosage Schedule for Treating Acute Mania and Maintenance Therapy

- Children under 12 year old: Not approved for use (see below under "Investigational Reports of Interest").
- Persons 12 years of age and older: Dosage must be individually regulated according to clinical response and serum lithium levels. As noted above, the pharmacokinetics of lithium carbonate make it necessary to administer the total daily dose in smaller doses administered three or four times daily if immediate release tablets or syrup is used or twice daily if controlled release capsules are used, to minimize risk of reaching toxic serum levels of lithium. (More detailed information on administering, titrating, and monitoring lithium in children and adolescents is found below.)

Dose Forms Available

- Tablets: 300 mg
- Capsules: 300 mg
- Controlled release tablets: 300 mg, 450 mg
- Syrup (lithium citrate): 8 mEq/5 ml (equivalent to one 300-mg tablet)

Titration of Lithium Dosage

Schou (1969) noted that early untoward effects, such as nausea, diarrhea, muscle weakness, thirst, urinary frequency, hand tremor, and a dazed feeling, may be caused by a too rapid rise in serum lithium levels. Lithium is also a gastric irritant. A low initial dose of lithium taken after meals, which slows absorption, and gradual increases in dose will often avert the development of these symptoms. When they develop, they usually subside spontaneously within a few days.

Serum lithium levels should be monitored twice weekly during the acute manic phase and until both serum level and clinical condition have stabilized. During maintenance therapy during remission, serum lithium levels and thyroid, kidney, and cardiac functions should be periodically monitored. The National Institute of Mental Health/National Institutes of Health (NIMH/NIH) Consensus Development Panel (1985) recommends that serum lithium levels be determined at intervals of 1 to 3 months and TSH and serum creatinine values be determined every 6 to 12 months. As there is less experience in long-term administration of lithium carbonate to children and adolescents than to adults, the author would recommend monitoring at the shorter recommended intervals—that is, determining the lithium level at least bimonthly and TSH and serum creatinine levels every 6 months.

Typically, doses of approximately 1800 mg/day will achieve the serum lithium levels of between 1 and 1.5 mEq/liter necessary to control symptoms during acute mania. During long-term maintenance serum lithium levels usually range between 0.6 and 1.2 mEq/liter; this usually requires a divided daily dose of between 900 mg and 1200 mg (PDR, 1990). Berg et al. (1974), however, reported that a 14-year-old girl and her father, who were both diagnosed with bipolar manic-depressive disorder, required daily doses of lithium as high as 2400 mg to achieve therapeutic levels.

The NIMH/NIH Consensus Development Panel (1985) notes that criteria for prophylactic use of lithium in children and adolescents do not yet exist, and so the preventive use of lithium must be based on clinical judgment. The risks versus the benefits for this age range are not yet firmly established, although available data suggest the potential problems are similar to those encountered in adults (NIMH/NIH, 1985).

The Use of Lithium Carbonate in Children under 12 Years of Age

The therapeutic dosages of lithium carbonate used in treating children over 5 years of age with various disorders do not differ significantly from those used in treating older adolescents and adults, and the principles of administration are essentially the same (Campbell et al., 1984a). This higher dose/body weight ratio may reflect the fact that higher renal lithium clearance may occur in children and adolescents compared to adults.

Weller et al. (1986) published a guide for determining the initial total daily lithium dose for prepubertal children 6 to 12 years of age. The guide and summary of how it is to be used are presented in Table 6.1. Lower initial doses should be used for children diagnosed with mental retardation or organicity (central nervous system damage) (EB Weller, personal communication, 1990).

The purpose of this guide is to reach therapeutic serum lithium levels (0.6 to 1.2 mEq/liter) as rapidly as possible using currently available tablet strengths without undue risk of reaching toxic serum levels. The authors administered lithium to 10 subjects diagnosed with manic-depressive illness and 5 subjects diagnosed with conduct disorder, following these guidelines. Thir-

Table 6.1.
Lithium Carbonate Dosage Guide for Prepubertal School-Age Children[a,b,c]

| Weight (kg) | Dosage (mg) | | | |
	8 A.M.	12 noon	6 P.M.	Total Daily Dose
>25	150	150	300	600
25–40	300	300	300	900
40–50	300	300	600	1200
50–60	600	300	600	1500

[a] From Weller EB, Weller RA, Fristad MA. Lithium dosage guide for prepubertal children: a preliminary report. J Am Acad Child Psychiatry 1986;25:92–95.
[b] Dose specified in schedule should be maintained at least 5 days with serum lithium levels drawn every other day 12 hours after ingestion of the last lithium dose until two consecutive levels appear in the therapeutic range (0.6–1.2 mEq/liter). Dose may then be adjusted based on serum level, side effects or clinical response. Do not exceed 1.4 mEq/liter serum level.
[c] Lower initial doses should be used for children diagnosed with mental retardation or organicity.

teen of the 15 subjects had serum lithium levels in the therapeutic range after only 5 days of lithium treatment. Side effects were reported to be minimal, primarily mild nausea, abdominal pain, polydipsia and polyuria, and an increase in preexisting enuresis. Most were transient, and none required discontinuation of lithium. As discussed above, some untoward effects of lithium appear to be related to too rapid increases in serum lithium level. It remains to be determined whether the use of the proposed lithium dosage guide will cause significantly more untoward effects or will increase their severity more than would a more gradual titration of lithium. In cases where very rapid control of symptoms is critical, however, it may be prove to be especially useful.

Investigational Reports of Interest

Lithium Carbonate in the Treatment of Mood Disorders (Mania, Bipolar Disorder), Behavioral Disorders with Mood Swings, and/or Patients Whose Parent(s) Are Lithium Responders

DeLong and Aldershof (1987) reported that 66% of 59 children diagnosed with bipolar affective disorder, 82% of 11 children with emotionally unstable character disorder, and 71% of 7 offspring of a lithium-responsive parent were treated successfully.

Varanka et al. (1988) treated with lithium carbonate 10 prepubertal children (9 males, 1 female) (mean age, 9 years 6 months ± 2 years; range, 6 years 9 months to 12 years 7 months). All 10 children were diagnosed with manic episode with psychotic features. Doses ranged from 1150 to 1800 mg/day (32 to 63 mg/kg/day). Therapeutic lithium levels of 0.6 to 1.4 mEq/liter were reached in all cases within 3 to 5 days. Substantial improvement was observed in all the children an average of 11 days (range, 3 to 24 days) after therapy was begun. All psychotic symptoms remitted, and mood normalized. The children became less irritable and destructive; their thought processes, motor activity, and attention spans improved remarkably. Untoward effects such as fatigue, diminished appetite, abdominal discomfort, nausea, urinary frequency, and tremor were infrequent and so mild that they did not necessitate discontinuation of lithium.

Lithium Carbonate in the Treatment of Disorders with Severe Aggression, Especially When Accompanied by Explosive Affect, Including Self-Injurious Behavior

In a double-blind placebo-controlled study of 61 treatment-resistant hospitalized children with undersocialized aggressive conduct disorder, both haloperidol and lithium were found to be superior to placebo in ameliorating behavioral symptoms (Campbell et al., 1984b). Optimal doses of lithium carbonate ranged from 500 to 2000 mg/day (mean, 1166 mg/day); corresponding serum levels ranged from 0.32 to 1.51 mEq/liter (mean, 0.993 mEq/liter), and saliva levels ranged from 0.81 to 5.05 mEq/liter (mean, 2.515 mEq/liter). The authors noted that lithium caused fewer and milder untoward effects than haloperidol did and that these did not appear to interfere significantly with the children's daily routines. There was also a suggestion that lithium was particularly effective in diminishing the explosive affect and that other improvements followed (Campbell et al., 1984b).

Vetro et al. (1985) treated 17 children aged 3 years to 12 years who were hospitalized for hyperaggressivity, active destruction of property, severely disturbed social adjustment, and not responding to discipline. Ten of the children had not responded to prior pharmacotherapy including haloperidol and concomitant individual and family therapy. Lithium carbonate was titrated slowly over 2 to 3 weeks to achieve serum levels in the therapeutic range (0.6 to 1.2 mEq/liter). Mean serum lithium level was 0.68 mEq/liter ± 0.30 mEq/liter. The authors reported that 13 of the children improved enough that their abilities to adapt to their environment could be described as good, and their aggressivity had been reduced to tolerable levels. Three of the four cases that did not improve had poor compliance in taking the medication at home. The authors also noted that these children usually required continuous treatment with lithium for longer than 6 months.

DeLong and Aldershof (1987) reported that rage, aggressive outbursts, and, interestingly, encopresis responded favorably to lithium pharmacotherapy in children with behavioral disorders associated with a variety of neurological and medical diseases, including mental retardation.

Lithium Carbonate in the Treatment of Attention Deficit Hyperactivity Disorder

Greenhill et al. (1973) and DeLong and Aldershof (1987) reported that lithium was not effective or worsened symptoms in the treatment of children with earlier equivalent diagnoses of ADHD.

7

Anxiolytics

BENZODIAZEPINES

Benzodiazepines, introduced into clinical practice in the early 1960s, were the most frequently prescribed drugs in the United States for the 12 years prior to 1980; in 1978 alone 68 million prescriptions for benzodiazepines were written for about 10 million individuals; over half of these were for diazepam (Ayd, 1980). Greenblatt, Shader, and Abernethy (1983) noted that by 1980 the trend toward increasing use of the benzodiazepines had reversed, perhaps subsequent to publicity about abuse of and addiction to the benzodiazepines. The abuse and addiction potential of the benzodiazepines continues to be of concern, and in 1989 New York State began requiring all prescriptions for benzodiazepines to be written on triplicate forms, as for other controlled drugs. It should be noted, however, that many experts feel that compared to other drugs of abuse, the dangers of benzodiazepines have been "greatly exaggerated" (Simeon & Ferguson, 1985). The American Psychiatric Association (APA) Task Force on Benzodiazepines in a summary statement noted that "overall, the APA Task Force found that benzodiazepines, when prescribed appropriately, are therapeutic drugs with relatively mild toxic profiles and low tendency for abuse" (Salzman, 1990, p. 62). Benzodiazepines are poor self-reinforcers of use and tend to be taken alone for pleasure rarely. An exception to this occurs among substance abusers. Benzodiazepine abuse is very frequent among alcoholics; cocaine, narcotic, and methadone abusers frequently abuse benzodiazepines as well. These groups use benzodiazepines to "augment the euphoria (narcotics and methadone users), to decrease anxiety and withdrawal symptoms (alcoholics) or to ease the 'crash' from cocaine-induced euphoria" (Salzman, 1990, p. 62).

Benzodiazepines appear to be prescribed to both older adolescents and adults for relief of anxiety and tension, muscle relaxation, sleep disorders, and seizures. In children, however, they are used primarily for treatment of sleep and seizure disorders and are used much less commonly for their anxiolytic and muscle relaxant qualities (Coffey et al., 1983).

Surprisingly little is known about the use of benzodiazepines in child and adolescent psychiatric disorders. In their important 1974 monograph, Greenblatt and Shader, after reviewing the use of benzodiazepines in children and adolescents, stated, "At present it is doubtful that the benzodiazepines have a role in the pharmacotherapy of psychoses or in the treatment of emotional disorders in children" (p. 88). More recently, the literature concerning their use in children has been reviewed by Campbell, Green, and Deutsch (1985) and Simeon and Ferguson (1985). Most published reports in the literature appeared in the 1960s and were open studies. Many of the studies were comprised of diagnostically heterogeneous subjects; results were discrepant. Diazepam and chlordiazepoxide were the drugs most frequently employed.

Coffey and her colleagues (1983) have emphasized that the infant has an immature liver and that the newborn's capacity for hydroxylation, demethylation, and especially glucuronide conjugation is limited until about 5 months of age, when the necessary liver enzymes reach and begin to exceed adult capacities. During childhood and until pubescence, enzyme activity levels may exceed those of adults, causing the rate of metabolism to exceed that in adults and necessitating more frequent administration of benzodiazepines than in adolescents and adults (Coffey et al., 1983).

At the present time, the psychiatric conditions occurring in childhood for which there is the most convincing rationale for the use of a benzodiazepine as the drug of choice are sleep terror disorder (pavor nocturnus) and sleepwalking disorder (somnambulism); however, these conditions are not usually treated with pharmacotherapy unless they are unusually frequent or severe. Both sleep terror disorder and sleepwalking disorder usually occur "during the first third of the major sleep period (the interval of nonrapid eye movement [NREM] sleep that typically contains EEG delta activity, sleep stages 3 and 4)" (APA, 1987, pp. 310–311). As benzodiazepines decrease stage 4 sleep, they theoretically might be of therapeutic value in these conditions. On the other hand, benzodiazepines are theoretically contraindicated in treating sleep disturbance in psychosocial dwarfism (psychosocially determined short stature), as they would further compromise nocturnal secretion of growth hormone, which occurs maximally during sleep stages 3 and 4, slow-wave sleep (Green, 1986). Reite et al. (1990) suggested that either 2 mg of diazepam or 0.125 mg of triazolam at bedtime may decrease the frequency of night terrors or somnambulism in children with severe cases.

If a benzodiazepine is used as a hypnotic, consideration of the drug's serum half-life is important. For example, both flurazepam (Dalmane) and triazolam (Halcion) are used for treating sleep disorders. Flurazepam is a long-acting benzodiazepine with a half-life (for it and its metabolites) of 47 to 100 hours. The manufacturer notes that this pharmacokinetic profile may explain the clinical observation that flurazepam is increasingly effective on the second or third night of use and, similarly, that after discontinuing the drug, both sleep latency and total wake time may still be decreased. Hence flurazepam appears to be most useful in persons with both significant daytime anxiety and insomnia. In contrast, triazolam, also an effective hypnotic, is a short-acting benzodiazepine with a relatively rapid onset of action and a half-life of 1.5 to 5.5 hours. This would suggest that triazolam is the drug of choice for sleep onset insomnia and is preferable in terms of less risk of any unwanted daytime sedation.

Werry concluded that if pharmacotherapy is necessary for certain childhood sleep disturbances, including insomnia, night waking, night terrors, and somnambulism, "probably" benzodiazepines are indicated and that they are "possibly" indicated for some kinds of anxiety (Rapoport et al., 1978b).

Klein et al. (1980) suggested that a supplemental low dose of a benzodiazepine (e.g., diazepam 5 mg) might be useful in treating residual anticipatory anxiety in school-phobic youngsters whose separation anxiety had been alleviated by treatment with imipramine.

Simeon and Ferguson (1985) reported that some overly inhibited children may show lasting behavioral improvement following brief (not exceeding 4 to 6 weeks) treatment with a benzodiazepine. They attributed the improvement to an interaction between disinhibition facilitated by the medication and social learning. Consistent with this, they noted that children and adolescents with impulsivity and aggression who were under significant environmental stress should not be treated with benzodiazepines, as the disinhibition could result in worsening of behavior (Simeon & Ferguson, 1985).

Most of the literature suggests that benzodiazepines usually worsen symptoms in psychotic children. In studies comparing dextroamphetamine, placebo, and chlordiazepoxide or diazepam in treating hyperactive children, chlordiazepoxide and diazepam were both less effective than dextroamphetamine, and placebo was rated better than diazepam (Zrull et al., 1963, 1964).

Contraindications for Benzodiazepine Administration

Known hypersensitivity to benzodiazepines and acute narrow-angle glaucoma are usually considered absolute contraindications.

Persons predisposed to substance abuse or alcoholism should be prescribed benzodiazepines with caution because they may cause physical and psychological dependence and also interact additively with sedative or hypnotic drugs.

Adolescents who are likely to become pregnant or who are known to be pregnant should rarely if ever be prescribed benzodiazepines, as there are suggestions of increased risk for congenital malformations. Also, maternal abuse of benzodiazepines may cause a withdrawal syndrome in the newborn (Rall, 1990). Simeon and Ferguson (1985) feel benzodiazepines are relatively contraindicated in children and adolescents with significant impulsivity, aggressiveness, and environmental stress (negative disinhibiting drug effects may occur).

Interactions of Benzodiazepines with Other Drugs

The most clinically important drug interactions of the benzodiazepines are associated with additive effects when combined with other sedative or hypnotic drugs, including alcohol (ethanol). Phenothiazines, narcotics, barbiturates, MAOIs, tricyclic antidepressants, and cimetidine (Tagamet) have been reported to potentiate benzodiazepines. The rate of absorption of benzodiazepines and the resulting central nervous system depression are both increased by ethanol (Rall, 1990). Benzodiazepines are relatively safe drugs, and even large overdoses are infrequently fatal unless taken in combination with other drugs (Rall, 1990).

Untoward Effects of Benzodiazepines

The most common untoward effects of benzodiazepines are manifestations of their being central nervous system depressants; oversedation, fatigue, drowsiness, ataxia, and confusion progressing to coma may occur at high doses. When anxiety is the target symptom, benzodiazepines should be administered in divided doses to minimize sedation.

"Paradoxical reactions," episodes of marked dyscontrol and disinhibition, have been reported in children and adolescents. Symptoms have included acute excitation, increased anxiety, increased aggression and hostility, rage reactions, loss of all control and going wild, hallucinations, insomnia, and nightmares.

Use of Benzodiazepines in Child and Adolescent Psychiatry

In general psychiatry, the benzodiazepines are indicated in the management of anxiety disorders or for the short-term relief of the symptoms of anxiety and the short-term treatment of some sleep disorders. They are also used to treat acute symptoms of alcohol withdrawal. Several manufacturers note that they are usually not indicated for anxiety or tension associated with the everyday stresses of life. The effectiveness of benzodiazepines in treatment lasting over 4 months has not been assessed by systematic clinical studies.

At the present time, there are no specific clinical guidelines for treating any of the childhood psychiatric disorders with benzodiazepines. If used, manufacturers' clinical recommendations for children should not be exceeded. Table 7.1 gives usual daily dosages for some benzodiazepines, an estimate of the serum half-life of the parent compound and/or its significant active metabolites, the youngest age for which the FDA has approved their use for any purpose, and, when available, suggested dosages for their use in child and adolescent psychiatric disorders.

It is recommended that the need for benzodiazepines be reassessed frequently and that they be discontinued within a relatively short period of time, usually within a few weeks.

Because of the relative paucity of information available on the use of benzodiazepines in children and young adolescents, some of the more important studies will be briefly reviewed below, but each benzodiazepine will not be considered individually.

Table 7.1.
Some Representative Benzodiazepines

Benzodiazepine (Trade Name) (Estimated Serum Half-Life)	Minimum Age Approved for Any Use	Usual Daily Dosage
Chlordiazepoxide (Librium) (half-life: 24 to 48 hr)	6 years	5 mg 2 to 4 times/day; max. 30 mg/day
Diazepam (Valium) (half-life: 30 to 60 hr)	6 months	1 mg to 2½ mg 3 to 4 times per day; titrate as needed and tolerated
Flurazepam (Dalmane) (half-life: 47 to 100 hr)	15 years	15 to 30 mg at bedtime
Triazolam (Halcion) (half-life: 1.5 to 5.5 hr)	18 years	0.125 mg to 0.25 mg at bedtime
Temazepam (Restoril) (half-life: 9.5 to 12.4 hr)	18 years	15 to 30 mg at bedtime
Oxazepam (Serax) (half-life: 5.7 to 10.9 hr)	6 years	Not established for children 6 to 12 years old; adolescents' usual dose is 10 mg three times daily to max. of 30 mg four times daily.
Lorazepam (Ativan) (half-life: 12 to 18 hr)	12 years	1 to 6 mg/day
Chlorazepate (Tranxene) (half-life: about 48 hr)	9 years	For children 9 to 12 years old, max. initial dose of 7.5 mg twice daily. Max. weekly increase, 7.5 mg. Max total dose, 60 mg.
Alprazolam (Xanax) (half-life: 12 to 15 hr)	18 years	See text

Chlordiazepoxide (Librium)

Investigational Reports of Interest

Chlordiazepoxide in the Treatment of Behaviorally Disordered Children and Adolescents of Various Diagnoses

Krakowski (1963) treated 51 emotionally disturbed children and adolescents aged 4 years to 16 years with chlordiazepoxide. Criteria for inclusion were the presence of anxiety (especially with coexisting hyperactivity), irritability, hostility, impulsivity, and insomnia. Nine children had concurrent individual therapy, and 7 received other medications, mainly antiepileptics. Chlordiazepoxide was administered initially in divided doses totaling 15 mg and individually titrated. Maintenance dosage for periods of up to 10 months ranged from 15 to 40 mg/day (mean, 26 mg/day). Twelve patients (23.5%) showed complete remission of psychiatric symptoms, and 22 (43.1%) improved moderately. Children with adjustment disorders were particularly likely to improve; specifically, 11 of 18 with conduct disorders, 2 of 3 with habit disturbances, and all 4 with neurotic traits showed marked or moderate remission of symptoms. Of 12 mentally deficient patients, 3 improved moderately and 3 improved markedly. Untoward effects were relatively infrequent and included drowsiness, fatigue, muscular weakness, ataxia, anxiety, and depression. They were alleviated to a satisfactory degree by dosage reduction in all but one case.

Kraft and coworkers (1965) prescribed chlordiazepoxide to 130 patients (99 males, 31 females) who ranged in age from 2 to 17 years (112 were between 7 and 14 years of age). The most common diagnoses were primary behavior disorder (50), school phobia (18), adjustment reaction of adolescence (17), and chronic brain damage (14). Most subjects had marked hyperactivity and neurotic traits. Dosage ranged from 20 to 130 mg/day and was administered in divided doses; 94 subjects (72%) received 40 mg or more daily. Moderate or marked improvement occurred in 53 subjects (40.8%). Forty subjects (30.8%) had either no or insignificant improvement, and 37 (28.5%) worsened. The diagnostic group showing the greatest improvement was school phobia (77%). Only 38% of the primary behavior disorder subjects and 41.2% of the adolescent adjustment disorder subjects improved to a moderate or marked degree. Of those with organic brain damage, 50% worsened, 28.6% showed minimal or no benefit, and none had an excellent response. Across diagnoses, symptoms of hyperactivity, fears, night terrors, enuresis, reading and speech problems, truancy, and disturbed or bizarre behavior were moderately or markedly improved in 40.8% of the 130 subjects. The authors concluded that chlordiazepoxide was effective in decreasing anxiety and "emotional overload" (Kraft et al., 1965). The authors also reported that 22 of the 130 had untoward effects of sufficient severity to interfere with treatment results and that 14 other subjects had milder untoward effects that were transient or responded to a lowering of the dose.

Breitner (1962) administered chlordiazepoxide 20 to 50 mg/day to over 50 juvenile delinquents between 8½ and 24 years of age. He reported the drug produced cooperativeness, released tension, created a feeling of well-being, and made the subjects more accessible to psychotherapy.

D'Amato (1962) treated 9 children aged 8 years to 11 years who were diagnosed school phobia with 10 to 30 mg/day of chlordiazepoxide for from 5 to 30 days. The children were also seen in psychotherapy. Only 1 child did not attend school regularly after the 2nd week of treatment. The author compared these 9 children with 11 other children aged 5 years to 12 years, also diagnosed with school phobia, whom she had treated over the 6 preceding years with psychotherapy only. Only 2 of these 11 children returned to school within 2 weeks, and 9 remained out of school for 1 month or longer. The author felt this strongly suggested that chlordiazepoxide was an effective adjunct to psychotherapy in mobilizing children with school phobia to return to school.

Petti and his colleagues (1982) treated with chlordiazepoxide 9 boys aged 7 years to 11 years who had failed to respond to 3 weeks of hospitalization and placebo. Subjects' diagnoses were conduct disorder (5, 3 of which had borderline features), personality disorder (3; 1 had borderline features), and schizophrenia (1). Verbal IQs on the Wechsler Intelligence Scale for Children (WISC) ranged from 71 to 110. Target symptoms were anxiety, depression, impulsivity, and explosiveness. The initial dose of chlordiazepoxide was 15 mg, in divided doses. Optimal dose was determined by individual titration and ranged from 15 to 120 mg/day (0.58 to 5.28 mg/kg/day). Children's ratings on optimal dose were compared to baseline ratings. Marked improvement was noted in 2 boys, improvement in 4, and no change or worsening in 3. The major improvements were increased verbal production, increased rapidity of thought associations, and a shift from blunted affect or depressed mood to a more animated appearance and feeling subjectively better. The authors noted that chlordiazepoxide had the most positive effect on children who were withdrawn, inhibited, anergic, depressed, or anxious. The child with schizophrenia had worsening of psychotic symptoms, and two children with severe impulsive aggressiveness had worsening of behavior; the authors suggest chlordiazepoxide's use may be contraindicated in such children (Petti et al., 1982).

Diazepam (Valium)

Investigational Reports of Interest

Diazepam in the Treatment of Children and Adolescents with Various Psychiatric Diagnoses

Lucas and Pasley (1969) in one of the few double-blind placebo-controlled studies of benzodiazepines in this age group administered diazepam to 12 subjects 7 to 17 years old (mean, 12.3

years) who were diagnosed as psychoneurotic (N = 10) or with schizophrenia (N = 2). All subjects were inpatients or in a day-care program. Target symptoms included moderate to high anxiety levels, highly oppositional behavior, poor peer relationships, and aggression. The initial dose of diazepam was 2.5 mg twice daily. The drug was increased until a satisfactory therapeutic response or untoward effects occurred. The maximum dose achieved was 20 mg/day. The study lasted 16 weeks, during which four sequences of drug and placebo were randomly used. Subjects were rated on 10 items: hyperactivity, anxiety and tension, oppositional behavior, aggressiveness, impulsivity, relationship to peers, relationship to adults, need for limit setting, response to limit setting, and participation in program. There was no significant difference between diazepam and placebo on any item for the 9 patients who completed the study (the 2 patients with schizophrenia and 1 other patient dropped out). However, when scores on all 10 items were combined, diazepam scored significantly better than placebo ($P < .05$). Clinically, though, the difference was not very apparent. Eleven of the 12 children participated in the study long enough to be rated on a global rating scale. Five subjects showed no change, 2 were somewhat more anxious, and 4 were definitely worse, with increased anxiety and deterioration in their behavior on diazepam as compared to placebo. From this study and their clinical experience with diazepam the authors concluded that diazepam was not clinically effective in reducing anxiety or acting-out behavior in children and young adolescents. Older adolescents appeared to react similarly to adults, and diazepam was felt to be useful in treating their anxiety.

Diazepam in the Treatment of Enuresis

Kline (1968) administered diazepam or placebo to 50 children and adolescents aged 3 years to 15 years with nightly enuresis, in a double-blind study. Organic uropathy and mental retardation were exclusion criteria. Initially 5 mg of diazepam were given in the morning and 10 mg at night. This was increased up to a total of 25 mg if no positive response occurred at a lower dosage. If the child had at most two wet nights weekly at time 4 weeks, he or she continued on the same condition for a total of 12 weeks, when the code was broken. If the subject had three or more wet nights nightly at time 4 weeks, diazepam was given on an open basis for weeks 5 through 12. After the code was broken, it was determined that at time 4 weeks the 28 children who were assigned to diazepam improved significantly more than those assigned to placebo ($P < .05$). Of the 28 on the drug, 22 became dry, 2 were wet one or two nights per week, 3 continued to wet six or seven nights per week, and 1 worsened. Only 1 subject of the 22 on placebo became dry. The others were unchanged, except for 1 who worsened. Of 21 children on placebo at time 4 weeks who were doing poorly and were switched to known diazepam, 12 became dry (Kline, 1968).

Diazepam, with its relatively low toxicity, may be a useful alternative to tricyclic antidepressants in those cases of enuresis where pharmacological intervention is clinically indicated.

Diazepam in Treatment of Sleep Disorders

In an open study, three children with somnambulism and pavor nocturnus and four children with insomnia were treated with 2 to 5 mg of diazepam near bedtime; all seven responded favorably (Glick et al., 1971). However, no controlled study of benzodiazepines in these disorders has yet been published.

Alprazolam (Xanax)

Investigational Reports of Interest

Cameron and Thyer (1985) successfully treated a 10-year-old girl with severe nightly attacks of pavor nocturnus with alprazolam. Initially 0.5 mg of alprazolam was given at bedtime for 1 week; the dose was increased to 0.75 mg nightly for the next 4 weeks, and then the medication was tapered off. Attacks of night terrors ceased on the first night and had not recurred once at follow-up 9 months later.

Pfefferbaum et al. (1987) used alprazolam to treat anticipatory and acute situational anxiety and panic in 13 patients aged 7 to 14 years who were being treated for concomitant cancer. Treatment was begun 3 days prior to and continued through the day of stressful procedures. Initial doses were 0.005 mg/kg or lower and were titrated upward based on efficacy and untoward effects. Total daily dose ranged from 0.375 to 3 mg (0.003 to 0.025 mg/kg). The authors noted that dose limits were fixed by the FDA as the study was done under an Investigational New Drug permit. Subjects were rated on four scales measuring anxiety, distress, and panic. The subjects' improvement was statistically significant ($P < .05$) on three scales and reached borderline significance on the fourth scale. Untoward effects were minimal, mild drowsiness being the most frequently reported.

Simeon and Ferguson (1987) administered alprazolam

openly to 12 children and adolescents aged 8.8 to 16.5 years (mean, 11.5 years) who were diagnosed with overanxious and/or avoidant disorder. After a 1-week placebo baseline period, to which none of the subjects responded, alprazolam was titrated individually over a 2-week period to maximum daily dosages from 0.50 to 1.5 mg. The total period of active treatment with alprazolam lasted 4 weeks. Seven of the 12 showed at least moderate improvement on several rating scales; no child worsened. Ratings by clinicians showed significant improvement of anxiety, depression, and psychomotor excitation; parents reported significant improvement of anxiety and hyperactivity on questionnaires; and teachers reported significant improvement on an anxious-passive factor. Improvement in the subjects' sleep problems was frequently reported by parents. The few untoward effects were mild and transient. Ferguson and Simeon (1984) reported no adverse effects of alprazolam on cognition or learning at therapeutically effective doses.

Simeon and Ferguson (1987) also noted that the children who responded best to alprazolam and who continued improved after the drug was stopped had good premorbid personalities and prominent symptoms of inhibitions, shyness, and nervousness. Children with poor premorbid personalities and poor family backgrounds tended to develop negative symptoms of disinhibition such as increased aggressiveness and impulsivity, especially at higher doses, and relapsed following drug withdrawal.

Klein and Last (1989) reported Klein's unpublished data from a clinical trial of alprazolam in children and adolescents whose separation anxiety disorder did not respond to psychotherapy. Alprazolam was clinically effective when administered to 18 subjects aged 6 years to 17 years for 6 weeks in daily doses of 0.5 to 6 mg/day (mean, 1.9 mg/day). Parents and the psychiatrist judged that over 80% of the subjects improved significantly, while 65% of the subjects rated themselves as improved.

AZASPIRODECANEDIONES

Buspirone Hydrochloride (BuSpar)

Buspirone hydrochloride is relatively new drug with anxiolytic properties that is not pharmacologically related to the benzodiazepines or barbiturates. Buspirone has been approved by the FDA for advertising as clinically effective for the management of anxiety disorders or the short-term relief of the symptoms of anxiety. It is not recommended for use in persons under 18 years of age as its safety and efficacy have not been determined in this age group.

Buspirone does not have cross-tolerance with the benzodiazepines and lacks anticonvulsant activity (Baldessarini, 1990). At therapeutic doses it is less sedating than the benzodiazepines. In addition, no evidence of physical or psychological dependence or a withdrawal syndrome has been reported, and it appears to have low abuse potential even by individuals at increased risk for drug dependency. It is not classified as a controlled (Schedule II) substance.

It has been reported that unlike benzodiazepines, which have an immediate anxiolytic effect, buspirone may take as long as 1 to 2 weeks for its antianxiety effect to fully develop (USPDI, 1990).

Indications in Child and Adolescent Anxiety
    Buspirone is approved only for treatment of anxiety disorders and the short-term relief of anxiety in individuals at least 18 years old.

Dosage Schedule for Treating Anxiety
- Children and adolescents: Not recommended.
- Persons 18 years old and older: Initiate treatment with 5 mg three times daily. Titrate to optimal therapeutic response by increases of 5 mg every 2 to 3 days to a maximum daily dose of 60 mg.

Dose Forms Available
- Tablets: 5 mg, 10 mg

Pharmacokinetics of Buspirone Hydrochloride

Peak plasma levels occurred between 40 and 90 minutes after an acute oral dose of buspirone. Average elimination half-life after single doses of 10 to 40 mg of buspirone is usually between 2 and 3 hours.

Contraindications for Buspirone Hydrochloride Administration

Known hypersensitivity to buspirone is an absolute contraindication.

It is recommended that buspirone not be used concomitantly with monoamine oxidase inhibitors.

Interactions of Buspirone Hydrochloride with Other Drugs

The knowledge of the effects of concomitant administration of buspirone and other drugs is very limited; hence buspirone should be used cautiously with other drugs. There are reports that patients receiving MAOIs have developed elevated blood pressure when given buspirone.

Untoward Effects of Buspirone Hydrochloride

The untoward effects most frequently reported by adults taking buspirone include dizziness (12%), drowsiness (10%), nausea (8%), headache (6%), insomnia (3%), and lightheadedness (3%). Of note, however, drowsiness and insomnia were reported to occur with approximately equal frequency in subjects taking placebo; hence these effects may not have been related to buspirone per se.

Investigational Reports of Interest

Buspirone Hydrochloride in the Treatment of Autistic Disorder

Because of its serotonin-inhibiting properties, Realmuto et al. (1989) treated four autistic children 9 or 10 years of age with buspirone 5 mg administered three times daily for 4 weeks, followed by a week-long washout period and 4 weeks of 10 mg twice daily of either fenfluramine or methylphenidate. Two of the four children showed improvement while on buspirone. None of the children experienced adverse untoward effects from buspirone.

Buspirone Hydrochloride in the Treatment of Overanxious Disorder with School Phobia

Kranzler (1988) reported a single case study in which a 13-year-old adolescent diagnosed with overanxious disorder, school refusal, and intermittent enuresis was administered buspirone. A previous trial of desipramine yielded some improvement but was discontinued at the patient's request because of untoward effects. Buspirone was begun at 2.5 mg three times daily. At 5 mg three times daily, some drowsiness occurred, particularly in the morning. Dosage was eventually stabilized at 5 mg twice daily. Scores on the Hamilton Anxiety Rating Scale dropped from 26 to 15 and stabilized, with improvement in phobic anxiety, insomnia, depressed mood, cardiovascular symptoms, and anxious behavior. The enuresis did not improve.

Other Drugs

ANTIHISTAMINES

Diphenhydramine (Benadryl) and hydroxyzine (Atarax, Vistaril) are the antihistamines most frequently used in treating emotionally disordered children and adolescents. Chronologically, they were also among the earliest drugs used in child and adolescent psychopharmacotherapy, and they remain among the safest medications yet employed.

Contraindications for Antihistamine Administration

Known hypersensitivity to antihistamines is an absolute contraindication.

Newborn infants (and hence nursing mothers), prematures, newborns, and infants are especially sensitive to the stimulating effects of antihistamines, and overdosage may case hallucinations, convulsions, or death.

Narrow-angle glaucoma, stenosing peptic ulcer, pyloroduodenal obstruction, and symptomatic prostatic hypertrophy or bladder-neck obstruction are relative contraindications. The anticholinergic effects of these agents may aggravate asthma.

Interactions of Antihistamines with Other Drugs

Diphenhydramine and hydroxyzine have potentiating effects when used in conjunction with other central nervous system depressants such as alcohol, narcotics, non-narcotic analgesics, barbiturates, hypnotics, antipsychotics, and anxiolytics.

Monoamine oxidase inhibitors prolong and intensify the drying effect (an anticholinergic action) of antihistamines.

Diphenhydramine (Benadryl)

Diphenhydramine has been used for over 35 years to treat psychiatrically disturbed children (Effron & Freedman, 1953). Although such use is still not approved for advertising by the FDA, it is reviewed here as some child psychiatrists continue to find it clinically effective.

Fish (1960) reported that diphenhydramine is most effective in behavioral disorders associated with anxiety and hyperactivity, but that it also could be useful in moderately (not severely) disturbed children with organic or schizophrenic (including autistic) disorders. A later study of 15 children, however, found no significant difference in behavioral improvement between diphenhydramine in doses of 200 to 800 mg/day and placebo (Korein et al., 1971).

Diphenhydramine is also effective as an anxiolytic, reducing anxiety before producing drowsiness or lethargy, in children up to about 10 years of age. However, it shows a marked decrease in efficacy when administered to older children; they respond like adults with untoward effects of malaise or drowsiness. Thus diphenhydramine is useful primarily as a bedtime sedative for older children with insomnia and/or nighttime anxiety (Fish, 1960).

Diphenhydramine has also been used to treat children with insomnia and/or children who wake up after falling asleep and have marked difficulty falling asleep again. Russo et al. (1976) compared diphenhydramine and placebo administered to 50 children aged 2 to 12 years who had difficulty falling asleep or problems with night awakenings. Diphenhydramine 1 mg/kg was significantly better than placebo in decreasing sleep-onset latency and decreasing the number of awakenings over a 7-day trial. Total sleeping time, however, was not significantly increased. Side effects were minimal.

Dosage Schedule for Treatment of Children and Adolescents

- Premature and newborn infants: Use is contraindicated.
- Infants over 20 pounds (9.1 kg) and older children: Begin with 25 mg dose and titrate upward with 25 mg increments for optimal response. A maximum dose of 300 mg/day or 5 mg/kg/day, whichever is less, is recommended.
- Maximum activity occurs in about 1 hour, and the effects last about 4 to 6 hours; thus the drug is usually administered three to four times daily.
- Young children appear to tolerate a higher dose per unit of weight than do adolescents and adults. Fish (1960) found a dose range of from 2 to 10 mg/kg/day, with an average daily dose of 4 mg/kg, to be most effective in treating her behaviorally disturbed youngsters.

Dose Forms Available
- Capsules: 25 mg, 50 mg
- Elixir: 12.5 mg/5 ml
- Injectable preparations: 10 mg/ml, 50 mg/ml

Untoward Effects of Diphenhydramine

The most frequent untoward effects are anticholinergic effects and sedation. Children do seem more tolerant to the sedative effects of diphenhydramine, but the clinician should still be alert to any cognitive dulling that may interfere with learning. Young children may sometimes be excited rather than sedated by diphenhydramine. It is cautioned that overdose may cause hallucinations, convulsions, or death, particularly in infants and young children.

Hydroxyzine Hydrochloride (Atarax), Hydroxyzine Pamoate (Vistaril)

Hydroxyzine is an antihistamine that is absorbed rapidly from the gastrointestinal tract. Its clinical effects usually become evident within 15 to 30 minutes after oral administration. It has been used widely as a preanesthetic medication in children and adolescents because it produces significant sedation with minimal circulatory and respiratory depression. It also produces bronchodilation; decreases salivation; has antiemetic, antiarrhythmic, and analgesic effects; and produces a calming, tranquilizing effect (Smith & Wollman, 1985).

Use in Child and Adolescent Psychiatry

One manufacturer states that "hydroxyzine has been shown clinically to be a rapid-acting true ataraxic with a wide margin of safety. It induces a calming effect in anxious, tense, psychoneurotic adults and also in anxious, hyperkinetic children without impairing mental alertness" (PDR, 1990, p. 1858). Hydroxyzine is approved for the symptomatic relief of anxiety and tension associated with psychoneurosis and as an adjunct in organic disease states in which anxiety is manifested. Its efficacy for periods longer than 4 months has not been demonstrated by systematic clinical studies.

Although not specifically indicated in the manufacturer's labeling, the sedation caused by hydroxyzine (as with diphenhydramine) has been utilized in the short-term treatment of insomnia and frequent night awakening in children.

Untoward Effects of Hydroxyzine

The most common untoward effects of hydroxyzine are sedation and dry mouth.

Dosage Schedule for Treating Children and Adolescents
- Children under 6 years old: Medication should be titrated individually and administered four times daily to a maximum of 50 mg/day.
- Children 6 years of age and older and adolescents: Medication should be titrated individually and administered three or four times daily to a maximum of 100 mg/day.

Dose Forms Available
- Tablets (hydroxyzine hydrochloride): 10 mg, 25 mg, 50 mg, 100 mg
- Capsules (hydroxyzine pamoate): 25 mg, 50 mg, 100 mg
- Syrup (hydroxyzine hydrochloride): 10 mg/5 ml
- Oral suspension (hydroxyzine pamoate) 25 mg/5 ml
- Intramuscular injectable (hydroxyzine hydrochloride): 25 mg/ml, 50 mg/ml

---

ANTIEPILEPTIC DRUGS

The use of antiepileptic drugs for treatment of psychiatric disorders in children and adolescents was reviewed by Stores in 1978. He concluded that "while some of the antiepileptic drugs show possibilities as psychotropic agents, their use in children with nonepileptic conditions such as behavior or learning disorders of childhood cannot be justified except as a carefully controlled research exercise" (p. 314).

At the present time, most clinical interest in this area appears to be centered upon the use of carbamazepine.

Carbamazepine (Tegretol)

Evans et al. (1987) attribute the increased interest in carbamazepine's use in child and adolescent psychiatry in part to both the increased awareness of the serious untoward long-term complications of neuroleptics and the finding that the untoward effects of carbamazepine are less formidable than initially thought. In particular, the serious blood dyscrasias, agranulocytosis and aplastic anemia are very rare. The risk of developing these disorders when treated with carbamazepine is five to eight times that of the general population; agranulocytosis occurs in about 6 per million and aplastic anemia in about 2 per million of the untreated general population (PDR, 1990).

Contraindications for Carbamazepine Administration

Known hypersensitivity to carbamazepine or tricyclic anti-depressants, a history of previous bone marrow depression, and the ingestion of an MAOI within the previous 14 days are absolute contraindications.

Interactions of Carbamazepine with Other Drugs

Carbamazepine has been reported to decrease the serum half-lives of haloperidol, phenytoin, theophylline, and other drugs.

Carbamazepine serum levels are markedly reduced by the simultaneous use of phenobarbital, phenytoin, or primidone.

Increased lithium serum concentrations and increased risk of neurotoxic lithium effects may occur when carbamazepine and lithium are used simultaneously, as carbamazepine decreases lithium renal clearance.

Recently the FDA advised that carbamazepine could lose up to one-third of its potency if stored under humid conditions such as in a bathroom. Supplies should be kept tightly closed and in a dry location.

Investigational Reports of Interest

Although approved only for treating certain kinds of seizure disorders and neuralgias, carbamazepine has been used to treat many psychiatric disorders. In adults, perhaps the best known of these is the treatment of lithium-resistant bipolar disorder. There is evidence that carbamazepine has acute antimanic and anti-depressive effects as well as longer-term prophylactic action in treating bipolar disorder (Post, 1987). Post (1987) notes that more severe and dysphoric mania and a rapidly cycling course, variables associated with a poor response to lithium, appear to correspond to better responses to carbamazepine. It has been suggested that the efficacy of carbamazepine in psychiatric disorders may be secondary to its hypothesized ability to inhibit limbic system kindling. Kessler et al. (1989) reported that three psychotic adults improved markedly when carbamazepine was substituted for their neuroleptic medication and suggested criteria to identify affectively ill patients who may have a primary or superimposed organic mood disorder and who might benefit from car-bamazepine.

There are many reports, particularly in the European litera-ture, of the use of carbamazepine on an open basis to treat children and adolescents with psychiatric disorders; however, fewer placebo-controlled studies have been published. In 1988 Pleak and his colleagues noted that carbamazepine was so frequently chosen to treat aggressive children and adolescents who did not respond satisfactorily to standard treatments that it had become "somewhat of a 'vogue' medication" (p. 502).

Remschmidt (1976) reviewed data from 28 clinical trials, 7 double-blind and 21 open studies, with a total of over 800 nonepileptic child and adolescent subjects who were treated with carbamazepine. Positive clinical results were found for target symptoms of hyperactivity or hypoactivity, impaired concentration, aggressive behavioral disturbances, and dysphoric mood disorders. In addition to these behavioral effects, Remschmidt suggested these patients also experienced positive mood changes, increased initiative, and decreased anxiety.

Groh (1976) reported on 62 nonepileptic children treated with carbamazepine for various abnormal behavioral patterns. Of the 27 who showed improvement, most had a "dysphoric or dysthymic syndrome," the most important features of which were emotional lability and moodiness, which were felt to cause most of the other behavioral abnormalities.

Kuhn-Gebhart (1976) reported symptom improvement in a large number of nonepileptic children who were treated with carbamazepine for a wide variety of behavioral disorders. The author reported that 30 of the last 50 patients treated showed good or very good responses, 10 had discernible improvement, 9 had no change in behavior, and 1 deteriorated. The author noted that the more abnormal the EEGs of these nonepileptic patients, in general, the better the response, that many of the good responders came from stable homes, and that poorer results were more frequent in subjects from unfavorable homes.

Puente (1976) reported an open study in which carbamazepine was administered to 72 children with various behavioral disorders who did not have evidence of neurological disease. Fifty-six children completed the study. The usual optimal dose was 300 mg/day (range, 100 to 600 mg/day). Carbamazepine was given for an average of 12 weeks (range, 9 to 23 weeks). Twenty symptoms were rated on a severity scale at the beginning and end of the treatment. Individual symptoms were present in as many as 55 and in as few as 2 of the 56 children. Over the course of treatment, a decrease in symptom expression of 70% or more occurred in 17 of 20 symptoms in at least 60% of the subjects. Interestingly, all 6 children (100%) with night terrors responded positively, as did 16 (94%) of the 17 children with other sleep disturbances. Anxiety, present in 47 children, improved in 34 (72%). Enuresis improved in 8 of 9 children (89%), and aggressiveness, present in 46 children, improved in 32 (70%). The most frequent untoward effects were transient drowsiness (20%), nausea and vomiting (4%), and urticaria (4%).

Pleak and his colleagues (1988) reported that adverse behavioral and neurological reactions developed in 6 of 20 male subjects, aged 10 to 16, who were diagnosed with various disorders but primarily ADHD and conduct disorder, and who were participating in an ongoing protocol evaluating the efficacy of carbamazepine in treating severe aggressive outbursts in child and adolescent inpatients. The untoward effects included a severe manic episode in a 16-year-old, hypomania in a 10-year-old, increased irritability, impulsivity, and aggressiveness and/or worsening of behavior in two subjects aged 14 and 15. Two 11-year-old boys developed EEG abnormalities, with sharp waves and spikes; one of these boys improved behaviorally but had his first two absence seizures in several years. The authors caution that patients must be monitored carefully for the development of adverse neuropsychiatric untoward effects.

Three additional cases of carbamazepine-induced mania have been reported in children (Reiss & O'Donnell, 1984; Myers & Carrera, 1989). Myers and Carrera (1989) speculated that when adverse behavioral effects such as irritability, insomnia, agitation, talkativeness, and prepubescent hypersexuality occur with carbamazepine administration, they may sometimes be symptoms of an unrecognized hypomania or mania.

Evans et al. (1987) have reviewed the use of carbamazepine in treating children and adolescents with psychiatric disorders including hyperkinesis, aggression, impulsivity, and emotional lability. They noted the lack of systematic, well-controlled studies. These authors also addressed the important issue of the behavioral toxicity of carbamazepine and noted that in their clinical experience in treating hyperactive and conduct-disordered children with carbamazepine, untoward effects on mood and behavior such as irritability, aggressiveness, increased hyperactivity, emotional lability, angry outbursts, and insomnia commonly occurred and sometimes resembled the target symptoms for which the drug was being prescribed.

Carbamazepine's status in treating child and adolescent psychiatric disorders still remains to be elucidated. While there are indications that it is being used by clinicians with increasing frequency to treat many neuropsychiatric disorders that have failed to respond satisfactorily to more standard therapies, and positive results have been reported, further research is necessary to determine its efficacy for specific disorders, and which symptoms or patients are most likely to respond well.

Phenytoin, Diphenylhydantoin (Dilantin)

Contraindications for Phenytoin Administration

Known hypersensitivity to the phenytoin or a related drug is an absolute contraindication.

Interactions of Phenytoin with Other Drugs

Acute alcohol intake may increase serum phenytoin levels while chronic alcohol use may decrease levels.

Tricyclic antidepressants may precipitate seizures in susceptible patients, necessitating increased phenytoin doses.

Many drugs have been reported to either increase, decrease, or either increase or decrease phenytoin levels. Obtaining serum phenytoin levels may help clarify the situation when necessary. Some drugs increasing phenytoin levels are alcohol (when acutely ingested), benzodiazepines, phenothiazines, salicylates, and methylphenidate. Some drugs decreasing phenytoin levels are carbamazepine, alcohol (with chronic abuse), and molindone.

Interactions of phenytoin and phenobarbital, valproic acid, and sodium valproate are unpredictable, and serum levels of the drugs involved may either increase or decrease.

Use of Phenytoin in Child and Adolescent Psychiatry

Three double-blind placebo-controlled studies that treated children and adolescents with phenytoin (diphenylhydantoin) reported it was not significantly better than placebo.

Lefkowitz (1969) reviewed some of the earlier literature in which phenytoin was administered, primarily on an open basis, to nonepileptic children with psychiatric disorders, with discrepant results. Lefkowitz compared the efficacy of placebo and phenytoin in treating disruptive behavior in male juvenile delinquents (mean age, 14 years 11 months; range, 13 years to 16 years 3 months) in a residential treatment center. Each group contained 25 subjects. Phenytoin or placebo was administered in doses of 100 mg twice daily for 76 days. Both groups showed marked reductions in disruptive behavior. Phenytoin, however, was not significantly better than placebo on any of 11 behavioral measures. In fact, placebo was significantly more efficacious than phenytoin in diminishing distress, unhappiness, negativism and aggressiveness. The author suggested that mild toxic effects of phenytoin such as insomnia, irritability, quarrelsomeness, ataxia, and gastric distress may have accounted for the superiority of placebo.

Looker and Conners (1970) administered phenytoin to 17 children and adolescents (mean age, 9.1 years; range, 5.5 years to 14.5 years) who had severe temper tantrums and suspected minimal brain dysfunction. Eleven subjects had normal EEGs, 3 had mildly abnormal EEGs, and 3 had abnormal EEGs, but no subject had clinical seizures. Subjects were placed on a 9-week double-blind placebo cross-over protocol, and phenytoin was titrated to achieve blood levels of at least 10 μg/ml; 12 of the 13 subjects who had final blood levels determined had adequate levels to suppress epileptic discharge. Scores on the Continuous Performance Test, the Porteus Maze Test, parent questionnaires for all subjects, and school questionnaires for 11 subjects showed no statistically significant differences between phenytoin and placebo. The authors noted, however, that there appeared to be some individual subjects who responded positively and rather dramatically to phenytoin.

Conners and colleagues (1971) treated 43 particularly aggressive or disturbed delinquent males (mean age, 12 years; range, 9 to 14 years) living in a residential training school with phenytoin (200 mg/day), methylphenidate (20 mg/day), or placebo administered for 2 weeks in a double-blind protocol. Although the authcrs note some limitations in their study, they found no significant difference between drugs and placebo on ratings by cottage parents, teachers, clinicians, and scores on the Rosenzweig Picture Frustration Test and Porteus Mazes.

Overall, while there are individual patients without seizure disorder who appear to benefit from phenytoin, as yet there is no convincing evidence from double-blind placebo-controlled studies attesting to the effectiveness of phenytoin prescribed for psychiatric symptoms.

OPIATE ANTAGONISTS

Opiate antagonists have been investigated in the treatment of mentally retarded persons with self-injurious behavior (SIB) (for review see Sokol and Campbell, 1988) and in the treatment of autistic disorder. Deutsch (1986) has given a theoretical ratio-nale for the use of opiate antagonists in the treatment of autistic disorder.

Naltrexone (Trexan)

Contraindications for Naltrexone Administration

The main contraindications are hypersensitivity, any liver abnormalities, and the concomitant use of any opiate-containing substances, legal or illegal.

Interactions of Naltrexone with Other Drugs

Serious adverse effects occur if narcotics are administered while taking naltrexone.

Use of Naltrexone in Child and Adolescent Psychiatry

Naltrexone, a long-acting, potent opiate antagonist, is a potentially useful agent in a subgroup of autistic children who have elevated endorphin (opioid peptides) levels.

Positive effects of naltrexone were reported in an open study of a severely disturbed 5-year-old autistic male who had no communicative language and exhibited severe withdrawal, stereotypies, aggressiveness, and hyperactivity (Campbell et al., 1986).

Campbell et al. (1989) administered naltrexone on an open basis to 10 hospitalized children aged 3.42 to 6.5 years (mean age, 5.04 years). The study lasted 6 weeks. Following a 2-week baseline, single doses of 0.5, 1, and 2 mg/kg/day were administered at 1-week intervals. Ratings were made 1, 3, 5, 7, and 24 hours after each dose, and 1 week after the last dose. Subjects showed diminished withdrawal at all three dose levels. Verbal production was increased at 0.5 mg/kg/day, and stereotypies were reduced following the 2 mg/kg/day dose. Symptoms such as aggressiveness and "self-aggressiveness" showed little improvement. The major untoward effect was mild sedation which occurred in 70% of the subjects. Laboratory measurements including liver function tests and ECGs showed no significant change from baseline. Overall, raters considered 80% of the children to be positive responders for some symptoms (Campbell et al., 1989).

Campbell et al. (1990) subsequently conducted a double-blind placebo-controlled study of naltrexone in 18 children aged 3 years to 8 years diagnosed with autistic disorder. The study consisted of a 2-week placebo baseline phase, random assignment to placebo or naltrexone for 3 weeks, and a posttreatment 1-week placebo phase. The initial naltrexone dose was 0.5 mg/kg/day; this was increased to 1 mg/kg/day if no adverse effects occurred. Nine children received naltrexone; the optimal dose was 1 mg/kg/day. Six subjects receiving naltrexone were rated moderate (5) or marked (1) improvement on Clinical Global Consensus Ratings, whereas only 1 child on placebo achieved a moderate rating and none was markedly improved. The difference was significant ($P = .026$). On the other hand, no reduction in symptoms occurred on the Children's Psychiatric Rating Scale or Clinical Global Impressions. Naltrexone did not appear to affect discrimination learning in an automated laboratory. The authors also reported that overall symptom reduction seemed better in older autistic children than in younger ones.

β-ADRENERGIC BLOCKERS

Propranolol (Inderal)

Although initially used primarily in controlling hypertension, angina pectoris, various cardiac arrhythmias, and other medical disorders, there has been considerable interest in propranolol's use in general psychiatry.

Propranolol is a nonselective β-adrenergic receptor blocking agent and is the most frequently used drug in this class. Propranolol and other β-adrenergic blocking agents reduce peripheral autonomic tone, thereby lessening somatic symptoms of anxiety such as palpitations, tremulousness, perspiration, and blushing. There is some evidence that the β-adrenergic blocking agents significantly reduce these peripheral, autonomic, physical manifestations of anxiety but may not affect the psychological (emotional) symptoms of anxiety (Noyes, 1988). Noyes (1988) concludes from his review of the literature that β-blockers are relatively weak anxiolytics compared to benzodiazepines and should be used for generalized anxiety disorder primarily in patients for whom the use of benzodiazepines is contraindicated.

In adults, propranolol has been investigated in treating anxiety disorders, including generalized anxiety, performance anxiety (stage fright), social phobia, posttraumatic stress disorder, panic disorder and agoraphobia, and episodic dyscontrol and rage outbursts (Hayes & Schulz, 1987; Noyes, 1988). It has also been used in treating schizophrenia. Propranolol is effective in the treatment of some antipsychotic-induced akathisias (Adler et al., 1986).

Contraindications for Propranolol Administration

Known hypersensitivity to propranolol is an absolute contra-indication.

Patients with bronchospastic diseases, cardiovascular conditions, diabetes, hyperthyroidism, or other medical disorders should have their medical status carefully reviewed (consultation with the physician providing care for the medical condition is recommended) before prescribing propranolol. Gualtieri and his colleagues (1983) cautioned that propranolol is contraindicated in children and adolescents with a history of cardiac or respiratory disease, who have hypoglycemia, or who are being medicated with a monoamine oxidase inhibitor.

Because significant depression has been reported as an untoward effect, it is not recommended for children and adolescents who are already depressed.

Interactions of Propranolol with Other Drugs

Propranolol may interact with many drugs. Three interactions among those most likely to be seen in child and adolescent psychiatric practice are (a) if used concomitantly with chlorpromazine, plasma levels of both drugs are increased over what they would be if used separately; (b) alcohol slows the rate of absorption of propranolol; (c) phenytoin, phenobarbitone, and rifampin accelerate propranolol clearance.

Untoward Effects of Propranolol

There are few reports of untoward effects in children or adolescents who received propranolol for psychiatric indications. Of greatest concern have been cardiovascular effects, which are detailed below. Propranolol has also been reported to cause significant depression of mood, manifested by insomnia, lethargy, weakness, and fatigue. Vivid dreams, nightmares, and gastrointestinal symptoms have also been reported.

Use of Propranolol in Child and Adolescent Psychiatry

There are few reports on the use of these drugs in psychiatrically disturbed children and adolescents.

Propranolol in the Treatment of Children and Adolescents with Brain Dysfunction, Uncontrolled Rage Outbursts, and/or Aggressiveness

Williams et al. (1982) administered propranolol to 30 subjects (11 children, 15 adolescents, 4 adults) with organic brain dysfunction and uncontrolled rage outbursts that had not responded to other treatments. The subjects had various psychiatric diagnoses, including 15 with the dual diagnoses of conduct disorder, unsocialized, aggressive type, and attention deficit disorder with hyperactivity; 7 with the dual diagnoses of conduct disorder, unsocialized, aggressive type, and attention deficit disorder without hyperactivity; 3 with conduct disorder only; 3 with intermittent explosive disorders; and 2 with pervasive developmental disorders. Thirteen had IQs in the retarded range, and 8 had borderline IQs. The authors reported that 80% of their subjects demonstrated moderate to marked improvement on follow-up between 2 and 30 months (mean, 8 months) later. Optimal dosages of propranolol ranged from 50 to 960 mg/day (mean, 160 mg/day). All untoward effects were transient and reversible with dosage reduction. Most of the patients were additionally treated with other medication: 13 subjects received anticonvulsants, 6 antipsychotics, and 3 stimulants; 21 had ongoing psychotherapy (Williams et al., 1982).

Kuperman and Stewart (1987) treated openly with propranolol 16 subjects whose mean age was 13.4 years (8 patients were 4 to 14 years old, 4 were between 14 and 17, and 4 were 18 to 24 years old). Seven subjects were diagnosed with conduct disorder, undersocialized aggressive type, 5 had infantile autism with varying degrees of mental retardation, 2 had moderate mental retardation only, 1 had borderline intellectual functioning, and 1 was diagnosed with attention deficit disorder. All subjects exhibited significant physically aggressive behavior that had not responded adequately to behavior therapy and/or psychotropic medication. Propranolol was begun at 20 mg twice daily and increased by 40 mg every fourth day until symptom improvement occurred or standing systolic blood pressure fell below 90 mm Hg, diastolic blood pressure fell below 60 mm Hg, or resting pulse fell below 60 beats per minute. The average dose of propranolol was 164 ± 55 mg/day. Ten patients (62.5%) were rated moderately or much improved, based on concurrence of ratings by parents, teachers, and clinicians. Responders and nonresponders did not differ significantly regarding age, sex, IQ, vital signs, or dosage. The authors noted that, although not significant, 6 of their 8 patients who were mentally retarded responded favorably, which is consistent with earlier findings in adults that suggest aggressive patients with suspected central nervous system damage respond best. Nonresponders as a group tended to develop bradycardia, which may have prevented them from reaching potentially therapeutic doses of propranolol. The authors additionally noted that before considering propranolol a therapeutic failure, a patient should receive the maximum therapeutic dose tolerated for at least 1 month. When propranolol is discontinued, it should be tapered gradually over a 2-week period to avoid rebound tachycardia (Kuperman & Stewart, 1987).

Two 12-year-old boys treated with propranolol for episodic dyscontrol and aggressive behavior showed marked improvement (Grizenko & Vida, 1988). Dosage was begun at 10 mg three times daily and gradually increased to 50 mg three times daily.

Famularo et al. (1988) reported that 11 children (mean age, $8^{1}/_{2}$ years old) diagnosed with posttraumatic stress disorder (PTSD), acute type, had significantly lower scores on an inventory of PTSD symptoms during the period they were receiving propranolol compared to scores before and after the drug. Dosage was begun at 0.8 mg/kg/day and administered in three divided doses; it was increased gradually over 2 weeks to approximately 2.5 mg/kg/day. Untoward effects prevented raising dosage to this level in only three cases. Propranolol was maintained at this level for 2 weeks and then tapered and discontinued over a 5th week. The authors emphasized that their subjects had presented in agitated, hyperaroused states and that propranolol might be useful during this particular stage of the disorder (Famularo et al., 1988).

At present, although there are some encouraging initial data, the use of propranolol and the β-blockers in children and adolescents must be regarded as investigational. In particular, propranolol's use in anxiety disorders remains to be elucidated.

α-ADRENERGIC ANTAGONISTS

Clonidine Hydrochloride (Catapres), Clonidine (Catapres-Transdermal Therapeutic System)

Clonidine is a centrally acting antihypertensive agent. The only therapeutic indication that has been approved by the FDA for advertising is treating hypertension in older adolescents and adults; its safety and efficacy in children have not been established.

Clonidine is an α-adrenergic stimulating agent that acts preferentially on presynaptic α_2 neurons to inhibit brain noradrenergic activity (Hunt et al., 1985). The authors note that the positive results in their studies with children diagnosed with ADHD gest that the norepinephrine system may be important in causing behavioral and cognitive abnormalities, in at least some children with ADHD.

Pharmacokinetics of Clonidine

Peak plasma levels of clonidine occur between 3 and 5 hours after ingestion, and plasma half-life is between 12 and 16 hours (package insert). Leckman et al. (1985), however, give different pharmacokinetic values for children and adolescents, stating that clonidine's half-life is about 8 to 12 hours in adolescents and adults, while in prepubertal children it is considerably shorter, approximately 4 to 6 hours. Between 40% and 60% of the drug is excreted unchanged by the kidneys within 24 hours after oral ingestion, and about 50% is metabolized by the liver (package insert).

Contraindications for Clonidine Administration

Significant cardiovascular disease and known allergic reactions to clonidine are relative contraindications. If clonidine is used in patients with such conditions, careful and frequent monitoring is required.

Children and adolescents with depressive symptomatology, past history of depression, or family history of mood disorder should not be given clonidine (Hunt et al., 1990).

Interactions of Clonidine with Other Drugs

Tricyclic antidepressants may decrease the effects of clonidine, necessitating higher doses.

The central nervous system depressive effects of alcohol, barbiturates, and other drugs may be enhanced by simultaneous administration with clonapine.

Interactions with additional drugs have been reported.

Indications in Child and Adolescent Psychiatry
There are no FDA-approved uses of clonidine in the treatment of psychiatrically disturbed children and adolescents. However, clonidine has been investigated in treating children and adolescents diagnosed with attention deficit hyperactivity disorder and/or Tourette's disorder who have not responded to standard treatments for these disorders. Studies of these uses and the doses employed by the researchers are summarized below for each of these conditions.

Dose Forms Available
• Tablets: 0.1 mg, 0.2 mg, 0.3 mg (all single scored)
• Transdermal Therapeutic System: Programmed delivery by skin patch of 0.1 mg, 0.2 mg, or 0.3 mg daily for 1 week

When a transdermal patch was used in treating subjects diagnosed with ADHD, Hunt (1987) found that its efficacy wore off and it had to be replaced in 50% of subjects after 5 days rather than the 7 days stated by the manufacturer. He also noted that to achieve the same degree of symptom control three of his eight subjects whose daily oral dose was 0.2 mg/day had to have their doses increased to 0.3 mg/day when clonidine was administered transdermally. Comings (1990), who has an extensive clinical experience with Tourette's patients, stated that he found that clonidine administered using a patch may work when oral clonidine is ineffective. Comings also found it convenient and useful to adjust the dose of clonidine by using scissors to cut the patch to the necessary size.

Discontinuing Medication

Clonidine should be gradually reduced over a period of 2 to 4 days to avoid a possible hypertensive reaction and other withdrawal symptomatology such as nervousness, agitation, and headache (package insert).

Investigational Reports of Interest

Clonidine in the Treatment of Attention Deficit Hyperactivity Disorder

Hunt et al. (1982) reported on an open pilot study in which clonidine 3 to 4 μg/kg/day was administered orally for 2 to 5 months to four children between 9 and 14 years of age diagnosed with ADDH. Improvement was noted by parents and teachers. The authors noted that distractibility often persisted, but the children were nevertheless more able to return to and complete tasks.

Hunt et al. (1985) conducted a double-blind placebo cross-over study of 12 children (mean age, 11.6 ± 0.54 years) who were diagnosed with ADDH. Ten children completed the study. Seven subjects had previously received stimulant medication; in four cases stimulants had been discontinued because of significant side effects. Clonidine was begun at 0.05 mg and increased every other day until a dose of 4 to 5 μg/kg/day (about 0.05 mg four times daily) was attained. Parents, teachers, and clinicians all noted statistically significant improvements on clonidine for the group as a whole. The best responders were children who had been overactive and who were uninhibited and impulsive, which, in turn, had impaired their opportunities to use their basically intact capacities for social relatedness and purposeful activity. During the placebo period, parents, teachers, and clinicians noted significant deterioration in overall behavior for the group, symptoms usually returning between 2 and 4 days after discontinuing the medication (Hunt et al., 1985).

The most frequent untoward effect seen in this study was sedation, occurring about 1 hour after ingestion and lasting 30 to 60 minutes. In all cases but one, tolerance to this effect developed within 3 weeks. Mean blood pressure also decreased about 10%.

Hunt (1987) compared the efficacies of clonidine (administered both orally and transdermally) and methylphenidate in an open study of 10 children diagnosed with ADDH, all of whom had ratings by both parents and teacher of more that 1.5 SDs above normal on Conners behavioral rating scales. Eight subjects (7 males, 1 female; mean age, 11.4 ± 0.6 years; range, 6.7 to 14.4 years) completed the protocol. Subjects received placebo, low-dose (0.3 mg/kg) methylphenidate, or high-dose (0.6 mg/kg) methylphenidate. Each of these conditions was randomized for a period of 1 week. All subjects then received an open trial of clonidine 5 μg/kg/day administered orally for 8 weeks. Eight subjects completed the open trial with positive results and were then switched from tablets to transdermal clonidine skin patch. Both clonidine and methylphenidate were significantly more effective than placebo, and clonidine in both dosage forms was as effective as methylphenidate (Hunt, 1987). Children reported they felt more "normal" on clonidine than on methylphenidate. Transdermal administration was preferred to oral administration by 75% of the children and their families, partly because the embarrassment of taking pills at school was avoided but also because it was more convenient. Local irritation from patches, however, at times prevented their use.

Hunt (1987) noted that in contrast to the stimulants, clonidine appears to increase frustration tolerance but does not decrease distractibility. He noted that an additional small dose of methylphenidate may be safely added to help focus attention and that this combination frequently necessitates a much lower dose of methylphenidate than would be required if it were the only drug used (Hunt, 1987).

In a recent review, Hunt and his colleagues (1990) explicated more specifically the differences between clonidine and methylphenidate in treating ADHD and their possible synergistic use in treating ADHD and suggested the subgroups of ADHD children for whom each treatment would be most useful. Stimulants (methylphenidate) improve attentional focusing and decrease distractibility, while clonidine decreases hyperarousal and increases frustration tolerance and task orientation.

The authors found that children with ADHD who respond best to clonidine often have an early onset of symptoms, are extremely energetic or hyperactive (hyperaroused), and have a concomitant diagnosis of conduct disorder or oppositional disorder. Such children often respond to clonidine treatment with increased frustration tolerance and consequent improvement in task-orientated behavior, more effort, compliance and cooperativeness, and better learning capacity and achievement. Clonidine also was efficacious in nonpsychotic inpatient adolescents with ADHD who were aggressive and hyperaroused (Hunt et al., 1990).

Unlike stimulants, clonidine does not directly improve distractibility; hence stimulants are preferable for mild to moderately hyperactive children with significant deficits in distractibility and attentional focus. The combination of clonidine and methylphenidate was found to be helpful for children who were diagnosed with coexisting conduct or oppositional disorder and ADHD and who were both highly aroused and very distractible (Hunt et al., 1990). The combined use of these drugs may permit the effective dose of methylphenidate to be reduced by about 40%, making it potentially useful for ADHD patients in whom significant hyperactivity, rebound symptoms, or dose-limiting side effects such as aggression, irritability, insomnia, or decrements in weight or height gain have occurred with stimulant treatment (Hunt et al., 1990).

At present, clonidine may be regarded as an investigational treatment for ADHD. However, it may eventually prove useful in treating, in particular, a subgroup of ADHD children who do not respond well to stimulants. Clonidine may also be considered as an alternative treatment for some ADHD children who have chronic tics or who develop side effects of sufficient severity as to preclude the use of stimulants (Hunt et al., 1985).

Clonidine in the Treatment of Tourette's Disorder

Cohen et al. (1980) reported that clonidine was clinically effective in at least 70% of 25 patients between 9 and 50 years of age diagnosed with Tourette's syndrome (TS) who either did not benefit from haloperidol or could not tolerate the untoward effects of that medication. Dosage was begun at 1 to 2 µg/kg/day (usually 0.05 mg/day) and gradually titrated up to a maximum of 0.60 mg/day. Most patients did best with small doses three to four times daily. Comings (1990) recommends a starting dose of 0.025 mg/day (one-fourth of a tablet) and sometimes found it necessary to administer as many as five divided doses daily for best results. He found it an excellent drug for the approximately 60% of his patients who responded and noted that it ameliorated oppositional, confrontative, and obsessive-compulsive behaviors and symptoms of ADHD when these were also present. On the other hand, Shapiro and Shapiro (1989) noted that in their experience clonidine was only rarely effective in treating unselected patients with tics and Tourette's disorder.

Cohen et al. (1980) delineated five phases of treatment response to clonidine:

Phase 1: Within hours or days, patients felt calmer, less angry, and more in control.

Phase 2: About 3 to 4 weeks after initiation of clonidine (usually coinciding with a therapeutic dose of 3 to 4 µg/kg/day [0.15 mg/day]), the patient recognized progressive benefits characterized by decreased compulsive behavior, further behavioral control, and decreased phonic and motor tics.

Phase 3: A plateauing of improvement started at about the 3rd month.

Phase 4: Five or more months after beginning, an increase in dosage up to 4 to 6 µg/kg/day (0.30 mg/day) of clonidine was needed to maintain clinical improvement.

Phase 5: Further tolerance to clonidine may occur at a dose considered too high to increase further.

A review of the use of clonidine in Tourette's disorder (Leckman et al., 1982) noted discrepant results among studies. The reviewers estimated that about 50% of subjects improved meaningfully. Behavioral symptoms showed the most improvement, and maximum benefit could take from 4 to 6 months. A minority of patients didn't respond, and a few worsened.

Leckman et al. (1985) reported a 20-week single-blind placebo-controlled trial of clonidine in 13 patients aged 9 to 16 years diagnosed with Tourette's syndrome. This was followed by a 1-year open clinical trial. The mean dose of clonidine was 5.5 μg/kg/day (range, 3 to 8 μg/kg/day) (0.125 to 0.3 mg/day). There was significant improvement in motor and phonic tics and associated behavioral problems. Forty-six percent of subjects were unequivocal responders, and 46% responded equivocally. Of interest is the fact that 9 of Leckman and colleagues' 13 patients also had an additional diagnosis of ADDH. As noted above, some children with ADHD have symptoms that also respond to clonidine.

Bruun (1983) has provided useful guidelines for prescribing clonidine for Tourette's disorder. She suggests initiating daily dosage at 0.025 mg twice daily for small children and at 0.05 mg twice daily for older children and adolescents. Medication is titrated upward gradually with increases of no greater than 0.05 mg/week; this slow pace often prevents untoward effects from interfering with the treatment. The usual optimal daily dose is between 0.25 and 0.45 mg. Doses above 0.5 mg/day may be required, but untoward effects (e.g., drowsiness, fatigue, dizziness, headache, insomnia, and increased irritability) become more troublesome. Bruun (1983) notes that drowsiness may occur at very low doses and suggests that no further increases in dosage be made until drowsiness subsides. Some patients note a decrease in beneficial effects 4 to 5 hours after their last dose, and treatment is usually more effective for all patients with total daily dosage administered in three or four smaller doses (Bruun, 1983).

Although presently not an approved treatment, there is evidence that some children and adolescents with Tourette's disorder respond favorably with significant symptom reduction when treated with clonidine. Clonidine may be regarded as a possible treatment for those youngsters with Tourette's disorder who have not responded satisfactorily or who have intolerable untoward effects to standard treatments.

BARBITURATES AND HYPNOTICS

At the present time, the barbiturates and hypnotics have little, if any, place in treating psychiatric disorders in children and adolescents. Today barbiturates, especially phenobarbital, are used in children and adolescents primarily for their antiepileptic properties. Behaviorally disordered children frequently may worsen when given barbiturates. As long ago as 1939, Cutts and Jasper administered phenobarbital to 12 behavior problem children with abnormal EEGs. Behavior worsened in 9 (75%), with increased irritability, impulsivity, destructiveness, and temper tantrums. The authors concluded phenobarbital was contraindicated in the treatment of such children. For sleep disorders, benzodiazepines, which are much safer to use, are now the drugs of choice.

Clinically, barbiturates have a disinhibiting and disorganizing effect on many psychiatrically disturbed children, including psychotic children. Cognitive dulling, an untoward effect of barbiturates, is also of major concern in children and adolescents. In adults, phenobarbital was found to decrease speed of access to information in short-term memory, and short-term memory itself was highly sensitive to phenobarbital levels (MacLeod et al,. 1978). The authors noted this could impair the ability of children and adolescents to maintain attention in the classroom and interfere with their learning new information.

Clinically, it is also important for the child and adolescent psychiatrist to remember that phenobarbital may contribute to disturbed behavior in some patients with seizure disorder in whom it is being used to control seizures. This is also the case in some younger children when phenobarbital is being used prophylactically (e.g., after febrile seizures). Some such children may show behavioral and cognitive improvement when they are switched to other antiepileptic medications.

References

Adler L, Angrist B, Peselow E, Corwin J, Maslansky R, Rotrosen J. A controlled assessment of propranolol in the treatment of neuroleptic-induced akathisia. Br J Psychiatry 1986; 149:42–45.

Allen RP, Safer D, Covi L. Effects of psychostimulants on aggression. J Nerv Ment Dis 1975;160:138–145.

Altamura AC, Montgomery SA, Wernicke JF. The evidence for 20 mg a day of fluoxetine as the optimal dose in the treatment of depression. Br J Psychiatry 1988;153(suppl 3):109–112.

Aman MG, Singh NN. Preface. In: Aman MG, Singh NN, eds. Psychopharmacology of the developmental disabilities. New York: Springer-Verlag, 1988:v–ix.

Ambrosini PJ. Pharmacotherapy in child and adolescent major depressive disorder. In: Meltzer HY, ed. Psychopharmacology: The third generation of progress. New York: Raven Press, 1987: 1247–1254.

American Medical Association. Drug evaluations. 6th ed. Chicago: American Medical Association, 1986.

American Medical Association. Drug evaluations. Chicago: American Medical Association, 1990.

American Psychiatric Association. Diagnostic and statistical manual of mental disorders. 2nd ed. Washington, DC: American Psychiatric Association, 1968.

American Psychiatric Association. Diagnostic and statistical manual of mental disorders. 3rd ed. Washington, DC: American Psychiatric Association, 1980a.

American Psychiatric Association. Diagnostic and statistical manual of mental disorders. 3rd ed., rev.) Washington, DC: American Psychiatric Association, 1987.

American Psychiatric Association. Tardive dyskinesia: Task force report 18. Washington, DC: American Psychiatric Association, 1980b.

American Psychiatric Association. Treatments of psychiatric disorders: A task force report of the American Psychiatric Association. Washington, DC: American Psychiatric Association, 1989.

Amery B, Minichiello MD, Brown GL. Aggression in hyperactive boys: Response to d-amphetamine. J Am Acad Child Psychiatry 1984;23:291–294.

Anderson LT, Campbell M, Grega DM, Perry R, Small AM, Green WH. Haloperidol in the treatment of infantile autism: Effects on learning and behavioral symptoms. Am J Psychiatry 1984; 141:1195–1202.

Arnold LE, Huestis RD, Smeltzer DJ, Scheib J, Wemmer D, Colner G. Levoamphetamine vs. dextroamphetamine in minimal brain dysfunction. Arch Gen Psychiatry 1976;33:292–301.

Assembly moves on clozapine controversy. Psychiatr News 1990;25(11):1, 13.

Ayd FJ Jr. Social issues: Misuse and abuse. Psychosomatics 1980;21(October suppl):21–25.

Baldessarini RJ. Drugs and the treatment of psychiatric disorders. In: Gilman AF, Rall TW, Nies AS, Taylor P, eds. Goodman and Gilman's The Pharmacological Basis of Therapeutics. 8th ed. New York: Pergamon Press, 1990:383–435.

Baldessarini RJ, Stephens JH. Clinical pharmacology and toxicology of lithium salts. Arch Gen Psychiatry 1970;22:72–77.

Ballenger JC, Carek DJ, Steele JJ, Cornish-McTighe D. Three cases of panic disorder with agoraphobia in children. Am J Psychiatry 1989;146:922–924.

Benfield P, Heel RC, Lewis SP. Fluoxetine: A review of its pharmacodynamic and pharmacokinetic properties, and therapeutic efficacy in depressive illness. Drugs 1986;32:481–508.

Bennett WG, Korein J, Kalmijn M, Grega DM, Campbell M. Electroencephalogram and treatment of hospitalized aggressive children with haloperidol or lithium. Biol Psychiatry 1983;12:1427–1440.

Berg I, Hullin R, Allsopp M, O'Brien P, MacDonald R. Bipolar manic-depressive psychosis in early adolescence, a case report. Br J Psychiatry 1974;125:416–417.

Bergstrom RF, Lemberger L, Farid NA, Wolen RL. Clinical pharmacology and pharmacokinetics of fluoxetine: A review. Br J Psychiatry 1988;153(suppl 3):47–50.

Berney T, Kolvin I, Bhate SR, et al. School phobia: A therapeutic trial with clomipramine and short-term outcome. Br J Psychiatry 1981;138:110–118.

Bernstein JG. Handbook of drug therapy in psychiatry. 2nd ed. Littleton, MA: PSG Publishing Co., 1988.

Bevan P, Cools AR, Archer T. Behavioural pharmacology of 5-HT. Hillsdale, NJ: Lawrence Erlbaum, 1989.

Biederman J, Baldessarini RJ, Wright V, Knee D, Harmatz JS. A double-blind placebo controlled study of desipramine in the treatment of ADD: I. Efficacy. J Am Acad Child Adolesc Psychiatry 1989a;28:777–784.

Biederman J, Baldessarini RJ, Wright V, Knee D, Harmatz JS, Goldblatt A. A double-blind placebo controlled study of desipramine in the treatment of ADD: II. Serum drug levels and cardiovascular findings. J Am Acad Child Adolesc Psychiatry 1989b;28:903–911.

Birmaher B, Greenhill LL, Cooper TB, Fried J, Maminski B. Sustained release methylphenidate: Pharmacokinetic studies in ADDH males. J Am Acad Child Adolesc Psychiatry 1989; 28:568–772.

Birmaher B, Quintana H, Greenhill LL. Methylphenidate treatment of hyperactive autistic children. J Am Acad Child Adolesc Psychiatry 1988;27:248–251.

Bowden CL, Sarabia F. Diagnosing manic-depressive illness in adolescents. Compr Psychiatry 1980;21:263–269.

Bradley C. The behavior of children receiving Benzedrine. Am J Psychiatry 1937;94:577–585.

Breitner C. An approach to the treatment of juvenile delinquency. Ariz Med 1962;19:82–87.

Bruun R. TSA medical update: Treatment with clonidine. Tourette Syndrome Assoc Newsletter, spring, 1983.

Burke P, Puig-Antich J. Psychobiology of childhood depression. In: Lewis M, Miller SM, eds. Handbook of developmental psychopathology. New York: Plenum Press, 1990:327–339.

Burke RE, Fahn S, Jankovic J, et al. Tardive dystonia: Late-onset and persistent dystonia caused by antipsychotic drugs. Neurology 1982;32:1335–1346.

Cameron OG, Thyer BA. Treatment of pavor nocturnus with alprazolam. J Clin Psychiatry 1985;46:504.

Campbell M, Adams P, Small AM, et al. Efficacy and safety of fenfluramine in autistic children. J Am Acad Child Adolesc Psychiatry 1988;27:434–439.

Campbell M, Anderson LT, Small AM, Locascio JJ, Lynch NS, Choroco MC. Naltrexone in autistic children: A double-blind and placebo-controlled study. Psychopharmacol Bull 1990;26: 130–135.

Campbell M, Green WH. Pervasive developmental disorders of childhood. In: Kaplan HI, Sadock BJ, eds. Comprehensive textbook of psychiatry. 4th ed. Baltimore: Williams & Wilkins, 1985: 1672–1683.

Campbell M, Green WH, Deutsch SI. Child and adolescent psychopharmacology. Beverly Hills, CA: Sage, 1985.

Campbell M, Grega DM, Green WH, Bennett WG. Neuroleptic-induced dyskinesias in children. Clin Neuropharmacol 1983; 6:207–222.

Campbell M, Overall JE, Small AM, et al. Naltrexone in autistic children: An acute open dose range tolerance trial. J Am Acad Child Adolesc Psychiatry 1989;28:200–206.

Campbell M, Perry R, Green WH. The use of lithium in children and adolescents. Psychosomatics 1984a;25:95–106.

Campbell M, Small AM, Green WH, et al. Behavioral efficacy of haloperidol and lithium carbonate: A comparison in hospitalized aggressive children with conduct disorder. Arch Gen Psychiatry 1984b;41:650–656.

Campbell M, Small AM, Perry R, Green WH. Pharmacotherapy in infantile autism: Efficacy and safety. In: Shagass C, Josiassen RC, Bridger WH, Weiss KJ, Stoff D, Simpson GM, eds. Biological psychiatry 1985. New York: Elsevier, 1986:1489–1491.

Campbell M, Spencer EK. Psychopharmacology in child and adolescent psychiatry: A review of the past five years. J Am Acad Child Adolesc Psychiatry 1988:27:269–279.

Carlson GA, Strober M. Manic-depressive illness in early adolescence. J Am Acad Child Psychiatry 1978;17:138–153.

Casat CD, Pleasants DZ, Schroeder DH, Parler DW. Bupropion in children with attention deficit disorder. Psychopharmacol Bull 1989;25:198–201.

Chatoor I, Wells KC, Conners CK, Seidel WT, Shaw D. The effects of nocturnally administered stimulant medication on EEG sleep and behavior in hyperactive children. J Am Acad Child Psychiatry 1983;22:337–342.

Ciraulo DA, Shader RI, Greenblatt DJ, Creelman W, eds. Drug interactions in psychiatry. Baltimore: Williams & Wilkins, 1989.

Clay TH, Gualtieri CT, Evans RW, Gullion CM. Clinical and neuropsychological effects of the novel antidepressant buproprion. Psychopharmacol Bull 1988;24:143–148.

Clements SD. Minimal brain dysfunction in children: Terminology and identification, phase one of a three-phase project. Washington, DC: US Department of Health, Education, and Welfare, 1966. (NINDB monograph no. 3.)

Coffey B, Shader RI, Greenblatt DJ. Pharmacokinetics of benzodiazepines and psychostimulants in children. J Clin Psychopharmacol 1983;3:217–225.

Cohen DJ, Detlor J, Young JG, Shaywitz BA. Clonidine ameliorates Gilles de la Tourette syndrome. Arch Gen Psychiatry 1980; 37:1350–1357.

Comings DE. Tourette syndrome and human behavior. Duarte, CA: Hope Press, 1990.

Comings DE, Comings BG. Tourette's syndrome and attention deficit disorder with hyperactivity: Are they genetically related? J Am Acad Child Psychiatry 1984;23:138–146.

Conners CK. Recent drug studies with hyperkinetic children. J Learning Disabilities 1971;4:476–483.

Conners CK, Kramer R, Rothschild GH, Schwartz L, Stone A. Treatment of young delinquent boys with diphenylhydantoin sodium and methylphenidate. Arch Gen Psychiatry 1971;24: 156–160.

Conners CK, Taylor E, Meo G, Kurtz MA, Fournier M. Magnesium pemoline and dextroamphetamine: A controlled study in children with minimal brain dysfunction. Psychopharmacologia (Berlin) 1972;26:321–336. (Reprinted in Kline DF, Gettelman-Kline R, eds. Progress in drug treatment. New York, Brunner/Mazel, 1975:700–715.)

Cooper GL. The safety of fluoxetine—an update. Br J Psychiatry 1988;153(suppl 3):77–86.

Crumrine PK, Feldman HM, Teodori J, Handen BL, Alvin RM. The use of methylphenidate in children with seizures and attention deficit disorder. Ann Neurol 1987;22:441–442.

Cutts KK, Jasper HH. Effect of benzedrine sulfate and phenobarbital on behavior problem children with abnormal electroencephalograms. Arch Neurol Psychiatry 1939;411:1138–1145.

d'Amato G. Chlordiazepoxide in management of school phobia. Dis Nerv Sys 1962;23:292–295.

deGatta MF, Garcia MJ, Acosta A, Rey F, Gutierrez JR, Dominiquea-Gil A. Monitoring of serum levels of imipramine and desipramine and individuation of dose in enuretic children. Ther Drug Monit 1984;6:438–443.

DeLong GR, Aldershof AL. Long-term experience with lithium treatment in childhood: Correlation with clinical diagnosis. J Am Acad Child Adolesc Psychiatry 1987;26:389–394.

Denckla MB, Bemporad JR, MacKay MC. Tics following methylphenidate administration: A report of 20 cases. JAMA 1976; 235:1349–1351.

Deutsch SI. Rationale for the administration of opiate antagonists in treating infantile autism. Am J Ment Deficiency 1986; 90:631–635.

Donnelly M, Rapoport JL, Potter WZ, Oliver J, Keysor CS, Murphy DL. Fenfluramine and dextroamphetamine treatment of childhood hyperactivity. Arch Gen Psychiatry 1989;46:205–212.

Dostal T. Antiaggressive effect of lithium salts in mentally retarded adolescents. In: Annell A-L, ed. Depressive states in childhood and adolescence. Stockholm: Almqvist & Wiksell, 1972:491–498.

Drug interactions and side effects index. Oradell, NJ: Medical Economics Co., 1990.

Dubovsky SL. Severe nortriptyline intoxication due to change from a generic to a trade preparation. J Nerv Ment Dis 1987;175:115–117.

Dugas M, Zarifian E, Leheuzey M-F, Rovei V, Durand G, Morselli PL. Preliminary observations of the significance of monitoring tricyclic antidepressant plasma levels in the pediatric patient. Ther Drug Monit 1980;2:307–314.

Duncan MK. Using psychostimulants to treat behavioral disorders of children and adolescents. J Child Adolesc Psychopharmacol 1990;1:7–20.

Effron AS, Freedman AM. The treatment of behavioral disorders in children with Benadryl. J Pediatr 1953;42:261–266.

Evans RW, Clay TH, Gualtieri CT. Carbamazepine in pediatric psychiatry. J Am Acad Child Adolesc Psychiatry 1987; 26:2–8.

Famularo R, Kinscherff R, Fenton T. Propranolol treatment for childhood posttraumatic stress disorder, acute type. Am J Dis Child 1988;142:1244–1247.

Ferguson HB, Simeon JG. Evaluating drug effects on children's cognitive functioning. Progr Neuropsychopharmacol Biol Psychiatry 1984;8:683–686.

Fish B. Drug therapy in child psychiatry: Pharmacological aspects. Compr Psychiatry 1960;1:212–227.

Fisher S. Child research in psychopharmacology. Springfield, IL: Charles C Thomas, 1959.

Flament MF, Rapoport JL, Berg CJ, et al. Clomipramine treatment of childhood obsessive-compulsive disorder: A double blind controlled study. Arch Gen Psychiatry 1985;42:977–983.

Flament MF, Rapoport JL, Murphy DL, Berg CJ, Lake CR. Biochemical changes during clomipramine treatment of childhood obsessive-compulsive disorder. Arch Gen Psychiatry 1987; 44:219–225.

Fleischhacker WW, Bergmann KJ, Perovich R, Pestreich LK, Borenstein M, Lieberman JA, Kane JM. The Hillside Akathisia Scale: A new rating instrument for neuroleptic-induced akathisia. Psychopharmacol Bull 1989;25:222–226.

Gadow KD. Children on medication: Vol. I. Hyperactivity, learning disabilities, and mental retardation. San Diego: College-Hill Press, 1986a.

Gadow KD. Children on medication: Vol. II. Epilepsy, emotional disturbance, and adolescent disorders. San Diego: College-Hill Press, 1986b.

Gadow KD, Poling AG. Pharmacotherapy and mental retardation. Boston: College-Hill Press, 1988.

Garfinkel BD, Wender PH, Sloman L, O'Neill I. Tricyclic antidepressant and methylphenidate treatment of attention deficit disorder in children. J Am Acad Child Psychiatry 1983;22: 343–348.

Geller B, Carr LG. Similarities and differences between adult and pediatric major depressive disorders. In: Georgotas A, Cancro R, eds. Depression and mania. New York: Elsevier, 1988:565–580.

Geller B, Cooper TB, Carr LG, Warham JE, Rodriguez A. Prospective study of scheduled withdrawal from nortriptyline in children and adolescents. J Clin Psychopharmacol 1987a;7: 252–254.

Geller B, Cooper TB, Chestnut EC, Anker JA, Price DT, Yates E. Child and adolescent nortriptyline single dose kinetics predict steady state plasma levels and suggested dose: Preliminary data. J Clin Psychopharmacol 1985;5:154–158.

Geller B, Cooper TB, Chestnut EC, Anker JA, Schluchter MD. Preliminary data on the relationship between nortriptyline plasma level and response in depressed children. Am J Psychiatry 1986;143:1283–1286.

Geller B, Cooper TB, Graham DL, Marstellar FA, Bryant DM.

Double-blind placebo-controlled study of nortriptyline in depressed adolescents using a "fixed plasma level" design. Psychopharmacol Bull 1990;26:85–90.

Geller B, Cooper TB, McCombs HG, Graham D, Wells J. Double-blind placebo-controlled study of nortriptyline in depressed children using a "fixed plasma level" design. Psychopharmacol Bull 1989;25:101–108.

Geller B, Cooper TB, Schluchter MD, Warham JE, Carr LG. Child and adolescent nortriptyline single dose pharmacokinetic parameters: Final report. J Clin Psychopharmacol 1987b;7: 321–323.

Geller B, Guttmacher LB, Bleeg M. Coexistence of childhood onset pervasive developmental disorder and attention deficit disorder with hyperactivity. Am J Psychiatry 1981;138:388–389.

Gittelman-Klein R, Klein DF, Katz S, Saraf KR, Pollack E. Comparative effects of methylphenidate and thioridazine in hyperkinetic children: I. Clinical results. Arch Gen Psychiatry 1976; 33:1217–1231.

Glick BS, Schulman D, Turecki S. Diazepam (Valium) treatment in childhood sleep disorder. Dis Nerv Sys 1971;32:565–566.

Green WH. Pervasive developmental disorders. In: Kastenbaum CJ, Williams DT, eds. Handbook of clinical assessment of children and adolescents. Vol. 1. New York: New York University Press, 1988:469–498.

Green WH. Psychosocial dwarfism: Psychological and etiological considerations. In: Lahey BB, Kazdin AE, eds. Advances in clinical child psychology. Vol. 9. New York: Plenum Press, 1986:245–278.

Green WH. Schizophrenia with childhood onset. In: Kaplan HI, Sadock BJ, eds. Comprehensive textbook of psychiatry. 5th ed. Baltimore: Williams & Wilkins, 1989:1975–1981.

Green WH, Campbell M. Advances in the psychopharmacology of childhood and adolescence. In: Noshpitz JD, ed. Basic handbook of child psychiatry. Vol. 5. New York: Basic Books, 1987:398–405.

Green WH, Campbell M, Hardesty AS, et al. A comparison of schizophrenic and autistic children. J Am Acad Child Psychiatry 1984;23:399–409.

Green WH, Deutsch SI. Biological studies of schizophrenia with childhood onset. In: Deutsch SI, Weizman A, Weizman R, eds. Application of basic neuroscience to child psychiatry. New York: Plenum Medical Book Co., 1990:217–229.

Green WH, Deutsch SI, Campbell M, Anderson LT. Neuropsychopharmacology of the childhood psychoses: A critical review. In: Morgan DW, ed. Psychopharmacology: Impact on clinical psychiatry. St. Louis: Ishiyaku EuroAmerica, Inc., 1985: 139–173.

Greenblatt DJ, Shader RI. Benzodiazepines in clinical practice. New York: Raven Press, 1974.

Greenblatt DJ, Shader RI, Abernethy DR. Current status of benzodiazepines (first of two parts). New Engl J Med 1983; 309:354–358.

Greenhill LL. Attention-deficit hyperactivity disorder in children. In: Garfinkel BD, Carlson GA, Weller EB, eds. Psychiatric disorders in children and adolescents. Philadelphia: WB Saunders, 1990:149–182.

Greenhill LL, Rieder RO, Wender PH, Bushsbaum M, Zahn TP. Lithium carbonate in the treatment of hyperactive children. Arch Gen Psychiatry 1973;28:636–640.

Grizenko N, Vida S. Propranolol treatment of episodic dyscontrol and aggressive behavior in children (letter to the editor). Can J Psychiatry 1988;33:776–778.

Groh C. The psychotropic effect of Tegretol in non-epileptic children, with particular reference to the drug's indications. In Birkmayer W, ed. Epileptic seizures—behaviour—pain. Bern: Hans Huber Publishers, 1976, pp. 259–263.

Gross MB, Wilson WC. Minimal brain dysfunction. New York: Brunner/Mazel, 1974.

Gualtieri CT, Golden R, Evans RW, Hicks RE. Blood level measurement of psychoactive drugs in pediatric psychiatry. Ther Drug Monit 1984a;6:127–141.

Gualtieri CT, Golden RN, Fahs JJ. New developments in pediatric psychopharmacology. Dev Behavi Pediatr 1983;4: 202–209.

Gualtieri CT, Quade D, Hicks RE, Mayo JP, Schroeder SR. Tardive dyskinesia and other clinical consequences of neuroleptic treatment in children and adolescents. Am J Psychiatry 1984b; 141:20–23.

Gualtieri CT, Wafgin W, Kanoy R, Patrick K, Shen D, Youngblood W, Mueller R, Breese G. Clinical studies of methylphenidate serum levels in children and adults. J Am Acad Child Psychiatry 1982;21:19–26.

Hamill PVV, Drizd TA, Johnson CL, Reed RB, Roche AF. NCHS growth charts, 1976. Monthly Vital Statistics Reports 1976; 25(suppl 3):1–22. (Health Examination Survey Data, National Center for Health Statistics Publication [HRA] 76–1120.)

Hayes PE, Schulz SC. Beta-blockers in anxiety disorders. J Affect Disord 1987;13:119–130.

Hayes TA, Logan Panitch M, Marker E. Imipramine dosage in children: A comment on "imipramine and electrocardiographic abnormalities in hyperactive children." Am J Psychiatry 1975; 132:546–547.

Herskowitz J. Developmental neurotoxicology. In: Popper C, ed. Psychiatric pharmacosciences of children and adolescents. Washington, DC: American Psychiatric Press, 1987:81–123.

Holzer JF. The process of informed consent. Bull Am Coll Surgeons 1989;74(9):10–14.

Horowitz HA. Lithium and the treatment of adolescent manic depressive illness. Dis Nerv Syst 1977;38:480–483.

Hunt RD. Treatment effects of oral and transdermal clonidine in relation to methylphenidate: An open pilot study in ADD-H. Psychopharmacol Bull 1987;23:111–114.

Hunt RD, Capper L, O'Connell P. Clonidine in child and adolescent psychiatry. J Child Adolesc Psychopharmacol 1990;1: 87–102.

Hunt RD, Cohen DJ, Shaywitz SE, Shaywitz BA. Strategies for study of the neurochemistry of attention deficit disorder in children. Schizophr Bull 1982;8:236–252.

Hunt RD, Minderaa RB, Cohen DJ. Clonidine benefits children with attention deficit disorder and hyperactivity: Report of a double-blind placebo-crossover therapeutic trial. J Am Acad Child Psychiatry 1985;24:617–629.

Jatlow PI. Psychotropic drug disposition during development. In: Popper C, ed. Psychiatric pharmacosciences of children and adolescents. Washington, DC: American Psychiatric Press, 1987:27–44.

Jefferson JW, Greist JH, Ackerman DL, Carroll JA. Lithium encyclopedia for clinical practice. 2nd ed. Washington, DC: American Psychiatric Press, 1987.

Jefferson JW, Greist JH, Clagnaz PJ, Eischens RR, Marten WC,

Evenson ME. Effect of strenuous exercise on serum lithium level in man. Am J Psychiatry 1982;139:1593–1595.

Jeste DV, Wyatt RJ. Understanding and treating tardive dyskinesia. New York: Guilford Press, 1982.

Johnston C, Pelham WE, Hoza J, Sturges J. Psychostimulant rebound in attention deficit disordered boys. J Am Acad Child Adolesc Psychiatry 1988;27:806–810.

Joshi PT, Capozzoli JA, Coyle JT. Low-dose neuroleptic therapy for children with childhood-onset pervasive developmental disorder. Am J Psychiatry 1988;145:335–338.

Joshi PT, Walkup JT, Capozzoli JA, Detrinis RB, Coyle JT. The use of fluoxetine in the treatment of major depressive disorder in children and adolescents. Paper presented at the 36th Annual Meeting of the American Academy of Child and Adolescent Psychiatry, Oct. 11–15, 1989, New York, New York.

Källén B, Tandberg A. Lithium and pregnancy. Acta Psychiatr Scand 1983;68:134–139.

Kashani JH, Shekim WO, Reid JC. Amitriptyline in children with major depressive disorder: A double-blind crossover pilot study. J Am Acad Child Psychiatry 1984;23:348–351.

Kaufmann CA, Wyatt RJ. Neuroleptic malignant syndrome. In: Meltzer HY, ed. Psychopharmacology: The third generation of progress. New York: Raven Press, 1987:1421–1430.

Kessler AJ, Barklage NE, Jefferson JW. Mood disorders in the psychoneurological borderland: Three cases of responsiveness to carbamazepine. Am J Psychiatry 1989;146:81–83.

Klein DF, Gittelman R, Quitkin F, Rifkin A. Diagnosis and drug treatment of psychiatric disorders: Adults and children. Baltimore: Williams & Wilkins, 1980.

Klein RG. Pharmacotherapy of childhood hyperactivity: An update. In: Meltzer HY, ed. Psychopharmacology: The third generation of progress. New York, Raven Press, 1987:1215–1224.

Klein RG, Landa B, Mattes JA, Klein DF. Methylphenidate and growth in hyperactive children: A controlled withdrawal study. Arch Gen Psychiatry 1988;45:1127–1130.

Klein RG, Last CG. Anxiety disorders in children. Newbury Park, CA: Sage, 1989.

Klein RG, Mannuzza S. Hyperactive boys almost grown up: III. Methylphenidate effects on ultimate height. Arch Gen Psychiatry 1988;45:1131–1134.

Kline AH. Diazepam and the management of nocturnal enuresis. Clin Med 1968;75:20–22.

Klorman R, Brumaghim JT, Salzman LF, Strauss J, Borgstedt AD, McBride MC, Loeb S. Effects of methylphenidate on attention-deficit hyperactivity disorder with and without aggressive/noncompliant features. J Abnorm Psychol 1988a;97:413–422.

Klorman R, Coons HW, Brumaghim JT, Borgstedt AD, Fitzpatrick P. Stimulant treatment for adolescents with attention deficit disorder. Psychopharmacol Bull 1988b;24:88–92.

Korein J, Fish B, Shapiro T, Gehner EW, Levidon L. EEG and behavioral effects of drug therapy in children: Chlorpromazine and diphenhydramine. Arch Gen Psychiatry 1971;24:552–563.

Kraft IA, Ardall C, Duffy JH, Hart JT, Pearce P. A clinical study of chlordiazepoxide used in psychiatric disorders of children. Int J Neuropsychiatry 1965;1:433–437.

Krakowski AJ. Chlordiazepoxide in treatment of children with emotional disturbances. N Y State J Medicine 1963;63: 3388–3392.

Kramer AD, Feiguine RJ. Clinical effects of amitriptyline in adolescent depression: A pilot study. J Am Acad Child Psychiatry 1981;20:636–644.

Kranzler HR. Use of buspirone in an adolescent with overanxious disorder. J Am Acad Child Adolesc Psychiatry 1988;27: 789–790.

Kuhn-Gebhart V. Behavioural disorders in non-epileptic children and their treatment with carbamazepine. In: Birkmayer W, ed. Epileptic seizures—behaviour—pain. Bern: Hans Huber Publishers, 1976:264–267.

Kuperman S, Stewart MA. Use of propranolol to decrease aggressive outbursts in younger patients. Psychosomatics 1987; 28:315–319.

Kutcher SP, Mackenzie S, Galarraga W, Szalai J. Clonazepam treatment of adolescents with neuroleptic-induced akathisia. Am J Psychiatry 1987;144:823–824.

Lader M. Fluoxetine efficacy vs comparative drugs: An overview. Br J Psychiatry 1988:153(suppl 3):51–58.

Leckman JF, Cohen DJ, Detlor J, Young JG, Harcherik D, Shaywitz BA. Clonidine in the treatment of Tourette syndrome: A review of data. In: Friedhoff AJ, Chase TN, eds. Gilles de la Tourette syndrome. New York: Raven Press, 1982:391–401.

Leckman JF, Detlor J, Harcherik DF, Ort S, Shaywitz BA, Cohen DJ. Short- and long-term treatment of Tourette's syndrome with clonidine: A clinical perspective. Neurology 1985;35: 343–351.

Lefkowitz MM. Effects of diphenylhydantoin on disruptive behavior. Arch Gen Psychiatry 1969;20:643–651.

Lena B, Surtees SJ, Maggs R. The efficacy of lithium in the treatment of emotional disturbance in children and adolescents. In: Johnson FN, Johnson S, eds. Lithium in medical practice. Baltimore: University Park Press, 1978, pp. 79–83.

Leonard HL, Swedo SE, Rapoport JL, Koby EV, Lenane MC, Cheslow DL, Hamburger SD. Treatment of obsessive-compulsive disorder with clomipramine and desipramine in children and adolescents: A double-blind crossover comparison. Arch Gen Psychiatry 1989;46:1088–1092.

Linnoila M, Dejong J, Virkkunen M. Monoamines, glucose metabolism, and impulse control. Psychopharmacol Bull 1989; 25:404–406.

Looker A, Conners CK. Diphenylhydantoin in children with severe temper tantrums. Arch Gen Psychiatry 1970;23:80–89.

Lowe TL, Cohen DJ, Detlor J, Kremenitzer MW, Shaywitz BA. Stimulant medications precipitate Tourette's syndrome. JAMA 1982;247:1729–1931.

Lucas AR, Pasley FC. Psychoactive drugs in the treatment of emotionally disturbed children: Haloperidol and diazepam. Compr Psychiatry 1969;10:376–386.

MacLeod CM, Dekaban AS, Hunt E. Memory impairment in epileptic patients: Selective effects of phenobarbitol concentration. Science 1978;202:1102–1104.

Mann JJ, Marzuk PM, Arango V, McBride PA, Leon AC, Tierney H. Neurochemical studies of violent and nonviolent suicide. Psychopharmacol Bull 1989;25:407–413.

Mattes JA, Gittelman R: Growth of hyperactive children on maintenance regimen of methylphenidate. Arch Gen Psychiatry 1983;40:317–321.

McBride MC, Wang DD, Torres C. Methylphenidate in therapeutic doses does not lower seizure threshold. Ann Neurol 1986; 20:428.

Meltzer HY, ed. Psychopharmacology: The third generation of progress. New York: Raven Press, 1987.

Meyers B, Tune LE, Coyle JT. Clinical response and serum neuroleptic levels in childhood schizophrenia. Am J Psychiatry 1980;137:1459–1460.

Molitch M, Eccles AK. The effect of benzedrine sulfate on the intelligence scores of children. Am J Psychiatry 1937;94: 587–590.

Molitch M, Poliakoff S. The effect of benzedrine sulfate on enuresis. Arch Pediatr 1937;54:499–501.

Molitch M, Sullivan JP. The effect of benzedrine sulfate on children taking the New Stanford Achievement Test. Am J Orthopsychiatry 1937;7:519–522.

Morselli PL, Bianchetti G, Dugas M. Therapeutic drug monitoring of psychotropic drugs in children. Pediatr Pharmacol 1983;3:149–156.

Myers WC, Carrera FIII. Carbamazepine-induced mania with hypersexuality in a 9-year-old boy. Am J Psychiatry 1989;146:400.

Naruse H, Nagahata M, Nakane Y, Shirahashi K, Takesada M, Yamazaki K. A multi-center double-blind trial of pimozide (Orap), haloperidol and placebo in children with behavioral disorders, using crossover design. Acta Paedopsychiatr 1982;48: 173–184.

National Institute of Mental Health/National Institutes of Health Consensus Development Panel. Mood disorders: Pharmacologic prevention of recurrences. Am J Psychiatry 1985;142: 469–476.

Neppe VM, Ward NG. The evaluation and management of neuroleptic-induced acute extrapyramidal syndromes. In: Neppe VM, ed. Innovative psychopharmacology. New York: Raven Press, 1989:152–176.

Newton JEO, Cannon DJ, Couch L, Fody EP, McMillan DE, Metzer WS, Paige SR, Reid GM, Summers BN. Effects of repeated drug holidays on serum haloperidol concentration, psychiatric symptoms, and movement disorders in schizophrenic patients. J Clin Psychiatry 1989;50:132–135.

New York State Department of Health. Safe, effective and therapeutically equivalent prescription drugs. 7th ed. Albany, NY: New York State Department of Health Office of Health Systems Management, 1988.

Noyes R. Beta-adrenergic blockers. In: Last CG, Hersen M, eds. Handbook of anxiety disorders. New York: Pergamon Press, 1988:445–459.

Nurcombe B. Malpractice. In: Lewis M, ed. The comprehensive textbook of child psychiatry. Baltimore: Williams & Wilkins, 1991:1127–1139.

Oxford English dictionary. Oxford; Oxford University Press, 1933.

Oxford English dictionary: A supplement to. Oxford: Oxford University Press, 1982.

Pangalila-Ratulangi EA. Pilot evaluation of Orap™ (Pimozide, R 6238) in child psychiatry. Psychiatr Neurol Neurochir 1973; 76:17–27.

Pare CMB, Kline N, Hallstrom C, Cooper T. Will amitriptyline prevent the "cheese" reaction of monoamine oxidase inhibitors? Lancet 1982:183–186.

Patrick KS, Mueller RA, Gualtieri CT, Breese GR. Pharmacokinetics and actions of methylphenidate. In: Meltzer HY, ed. Psychopharmacology: The third generation of progress. New York: Raven Press, 1987:1387–1395.

Pelham WE, Bender ME, Caddell J, Booth S, Moorer SH. Methylphenidate and children with attention deficit disorder. Arch Gen Psychiatry 1985;42:948–952.

Pelham WE, Sturges J, Hoza JA, Schmidt C, Bijlsma JJ, Milich R, Moorer S. Sustained release and standard methylphenidate effects on cognitive and social behavior in children with attention deficit disorder. Pediatrics 1987;80:491–501.

Perry R, Campbell M, Adams P, et al. Long-term efficacy of haloperidol in autistic children: Continuous versus discontinuous drug administration. J Am Acad Child Adolesc Psychiatry 1989;28:87–92.

Perry R, Campbell M, Green WH, et al. Neuroleptic-related dyskinesias in autistic children: A prospective study. Psychopharmacol Bull 1985;21:140–143.

Perry R, Campbell M, Grega DM, Anderson L. Saliva lithium levels in children: Their use in monitoring serum lithium levels and lithium side effects. J Clin Psychopharmacol 1984;4:199–202.

Pesikoff RB, Davis PC. Treatment of pavor nocturnus and somnambulism in children. Am J Psychiatry 1971;128:778–781.

Petti, TA, Fish B, Shapiro T, Cohen IL, Campbell M. Effects of chlordiazepoxide in disturbed children: A pilot study. J Clin Psychopharmacol 1982;2:270–273.

Pfefferbaum G, Overall JE, Boren HA, Frankel LS, Sullivan

MR, Johnson K. Alprazolam in the treatment of anticipatory and acute situational anxiety in children with cancer. J Am Acad Child Adolesc Psychiatry 1987;26;532–535.

Physicians' desk reference. 44th ed. Oradell, NJ: Medical Economics Co., 1990.

Platt JE, Campbell M, Green WH, Grega DM. Cognitive effect of lithium carbonate and haloperidol in treatment resistant aggressive children. Arch Gen Psychiatry 1984;41:657–662.

Pleak RR, Birmaher B, Gavrilescu A, Abichandani C, Williams DT. Mania and neuropsychiatric excitation following carbamazepine. J Am Acad Child Adolesc Psychiatry 1988;27: 500–503.

Pool D, Bloom W, Mielke DH, Roniger JJ, Gallant DM. A controlled evaluation of loxitane in seventy-five adolescent schizophrenic patients. Curr Ther Res 1976;19:99–104.

Popper C. Medical unknown and ethical consent: Prescribing psychotropic medications for children in the face of uncertainty. In: Popper C, ed. Psychiatric pharmacosciences of children and adolescents. Washington, DC: American Psychiatric Press, 1987a.

Popper C, ed. Psychiatric pharmacosciences of children and adolescents. Washington, DC: American Psychiatric Press, 1987b.

Post RM. Mechanisms of action of carbamazepine and related anticonvulsants in affective illness. In: Meltzer HY, ed. Psychopharmacology: The third generation of progress. New York: Raven Press, 1987:567–576.

Potter WZ, Calil HM, Sutfin TA, Zavadil III AP, Jusko WJ, Rapoport J, Goodwin FK. Active metabolites of imipramine and desipramine in man. Clin Pharmacol Ther 1982;31:393–401.

Poussaint AF, Ditman KS. A controlled study of imipramine (tofranil) in the treatment of childhood enuresis. J Pediatr 1965; 67:283–290.

Preskorn SH, Bupp SJ, Weller EB, Weller RA. Plasma levels of imipramine and metabolites in 68 hospitalized children. J Am Acad Child Adolesc Psychiatry, 1989a;28:373–375.

Preskorn SH, Jerkovich GS, Beber JH, Widener P. Therapeutic drug monitoring of tricyclic antidepressants: A standard of care issue. Psychopharmacol Bull 1989b:25:281–284.

Preskorn SH, Weller E, Jerkovich G, Hughes CW, Weller R. Depression in children: Concentration dependent CNS toxicity of tricyclic antidepressants. Psychopharmacol Bull 1988;24: 275–279.

Prien RF. Methods and models for placebo use in pharmacotherapeutic trials. Psychopharmacol Bull 1988;24:4–8.

Psychopharmacology Bulletin. Special Issue: Pharmacotherapy of Children. US Department of Health, Education, and Welfare pub. no. (HSM) 73-9002, 1973.

Puente RM. The use of carbamazepine in the treatment of behavioural disorders in children. In: Birkmayer W, ed. Epileptic seizures—behaviour—pain. Bern: Hans Huber Publishers, 1976: 243–252.

Puig-Antich J. Affective disorders in children and adolescents: Diagnostic validity and psychobiology. In: Meltzer HY, ed. Psychopharmacology: The third generation of progress. New York: Raven Press, 1987:843–859.

Puig-Antich J, Perel JM, Lupatkin W, et al. Imipramine in prepubertal major depressive disorders. Arch Gen Psychiatry 1987;44:81–89.

Rall TW. Hypnotics and sedatives; ethanol. In: Gilman AF, Rall TW, Nies AS, Taylor P, eds. Goodman and Gilman's the pharmacological basis of therapeutics. 8th ed. New York: Pergamon Press, 1990:345–382.

Rapoport JL, Buchsbaum MS, Weingartner H, Zahn TP, Ludlow C, Mikkelsen EJ. Dextroamphetamine: Its cognitive and behavioral effects in normal and hyperactive boys and normal men. Arch Gen Psychiatry 1980a;37:933–943.

Rapoport JL, Buchsbaum MS, Zahn TP, Weingartner H, Ludlow C, Mikkelsen EJ. Dextroamphetamine: Cognitive and behavioral effects in normal prepubertal boys. Science 1978a;199: 560–563.

Rapoport JL, Mikkelsen EJ. Antidepressants. In: Werry JS, ed. Pediatric psychopharmacology: The use of behavior modifying drugs in children. New York: Brunner/Mazel, 1978:208–233.

Rapoport JL, Mikkelsen EJ, Werry JS. Antimanic, antianxiety, hallucinogenic and miscellaneous drugs. In: Werry JS, ed. Pediatric psychopharmacology: The use of behavior modifying drugs in children. New York: Brunner/Mazel, 1978b:316–355.

Rapoport JL, Mikkelsen EJ, Zavadil A, Nee L, Gruenau C, Mendelson W, Gillin JC. Childhood enuresis: Psychopathology, plasma tricyclic concentration and antienuretic effect. Arch Gen Psychiatry 1980b;37:1146–1152.

Rapoport JL, Quinn PO, Bradbard G, Riddle M, Brooks E. Imipramine and methylphenidate treatment of hyperactive boys. Arch Gen Psychiatry 1974;30:789–798.

Rating scales and assessment instruments for use in pediatric psychopharmacology research. Psychopharmacol Bull 1985;21: 713–1124.

Realmuto GM, August GJ, Garfinkel BD. Clinical effect of buspirone in autistic children. J Clin Psychopharmacol 1989;9: 122–125.

Realmuto GM, Erickson WD, Yellin AM, Hopwood JH, Greenberg LM. Clinical comparison of thiothixene and thioridazine in schizophrenic adolescents. Am J Psychiatry 1984;141:440–442.

Reisberg B, Gershon S. Side effects associated with lithium therapy. Arch Gen Psychiatry 1979;36:879–887.

Reiss AL, O'Donnell DJ. Carbamazepine-induced mania in two children: Case report. J Clin Psychiatry 1984;45:272–274.

Reite ML, Nagel KE, Ruddy JR. Concise guide to evaluation and management of sleep disorders. Washington, DC: American Psychiatric Press, 1990.

Remschmidt H. The psychotropic effect of carbamazepine in non-epileptic patients, with particular reference to problems posed by clinical studies in children with behavioural disorders. In: Birkmayer W, ed. Epileptic seizures—behaviour—pain. Bern: Hans Huber Publishers, 1976:253–258.

Riddle MA, Hardin MT, Cho SC, Woolston JL, Leckman JF. Desipramine treatment of boys with attention-deficit hyperactivity disorder and tics: Preliminary clinical experiences. J Am Acad Child Adolesc Psychiatry 1988;27:811–814.

Riddle MA, Hardin MT, King R, Scahill L, Woolston JL. Fluoxetine treatment of children and adolescents with Tourette's and obsessive compulsive disorders: Preliminary clinical experience. J Am Acad Child Adolesc Psychiatry 1990;29:45–48.

Rifkin A, Quitkin F, Klein DF. Akinesia: A poorly recognized drug-induced extrapyramidal behavior disorder. Arch Gen Psychiatry 1975;32:672–674.

Ritvo ER, Freeman BJ, Geller E, Yuwiler A. Effects of fenfluramine on 14 outpatients with the syndrome of autism. J Am Acad Child Psychiatry 1983;22:549–558.

Rivera-Calimlim L, Griesbach PH, Perlmutter R. Plasma chlorpromazine concentrations in children with behavioral disorders and mental illness. Clin Pharmacol Ther 1979;26:114–121.

Rivera-Calimlim L, Nasrallah H, Strauss J, Lasagna L. Clinical response and plasma levels: Effect of dose, dosage schedules, and drug interactions on plasma chlorpromazine levels. Am J Psychiatry 1976;133:646–652.

Rosse RB, Giese AA, Deutsch SI, Morihisa JM. Laboratory diagnostic testing in psychiatry. Washington, DC: American Psychiatric Press, 1989.

Rudorfer MV, Potter WZ. Pharmacokinetics of antidepressants. In: Meltzer HY, ed. Psychopharmacology: The third generation of progress. New York: Raven Press, 1987:1353–1363.

Russo RM, Gururaj VJ, Allen JE. The effectiveness of diphenhydramine HCl in pediatric sleep disorders. J Clin Pharmacol 1976;4:284–288.

Ryan ND. Heterocyclic antidepressants in children and adolescents. J Child Adolesc Psychopharmacol 1990;1:21–31.

Ryan ND, Meyer V, Dachille S, Mazzie D, Puig-Antich J. Lithium antidepressant augmentation in TCA-refractory depression in adolescents. J Acad Child Adolesc Psychiatry 1988a;27: 371–376.

Ryan ND, Puig-Antich J, Cooper T, et al. Imipramine in adolescent major depression: Plasma level and clinical response. Acta Psychiatr Scand 1986;73:275–288.

Ryan ND, Puig-Antich J, Cooper TB, Rabinovich H, Ambrosini P, Fried J, Davies M, Torres D, Suckow RF. Relative safety of single versus divided dose imipramine in adolescent major depression. J Am Acad Child Adolesc Psychiatry 1987; 26:400–406.

Ryan ND, Puig-Antich J, Rabinovich H, et al. MAOIs in adolescent major depression unresponsive to tricyclic antidepressants. J Am Acad Child Adolesc Psychiatry 1988;27:755–758.

Safer D, Allen RP, Barr E. Depression of growth in hyperactive children on stimulant drugs. New Engl J Med 1972;287:217–220.

Sallee F, Stiller R, Perel J, Bates T. Oral pemoline kinetics in hyperactive children. Clin Pharmacol Ther 1985;37:606–609.

Sallee FR, Stiller RL, Perel JM, Everett G. Pemoline-induced abnormal involuntary movements. J Clin Psychopharmacol 1989; 9:125–129.

Salzman C. Benzodiazepine dependency: Summary of the APA task force on benzodiazepines. Psychopharmacol Bull 1990; 26:61–62.

Saraf KR, Klein DF, Gittelman-Klein R, Groff S. Imipramine side effects in children. Psychopharmacologia (Berlin) 1974;37: 265–274.

Schooler NR, Kane JM. Research diagnoses for tardive dyskinesia. Arch Gen Psychiatry 1982;38:486–487.

Schou M. Lithium: Elimination rate, dosage, control, poisoning, goiter, mode of action. Acta Psychiatr Scand 1969; 207(suppl):49–59.

Schroeder JS, Mullin AV, Elliott GR, Steiner H, Nichols M, Gordon A, Paulow M. Cardiovascular effects of desipramine in children. J Am Acad Child Adolesc Psychiatry 1989;28:376–379.

Shapiro AK, Shapiro E. Controlled study of pimozide vs. placebo in Tourette's syndrome. J Am Acad Child Psychiatry 1984;23:161–173.

Shapiro AK, Shapiro E. Do stimulants provoke, cause, or exacerbate tics and Tourette syndrome? Compr Psychiatry 1981; 22:265–273.

Shapiro AK, Shapiro E. Tic disorders. In: Kaplan HI, Sadock BJ, eds. Comprehensive textbook of psychiatry. 5th ed. Baltimore: Williams & Wilkins, 1989:1865–1878.

Shapiro AK, Shapiro E, Eisenkraft GJ. Treatment of Gilles de la Tourette syndrome with pimozide. Am J Psychiatry 1983;140: 1183–1186.

Sheard MH. Lithium in the treatment of aggression. J Nerv Ment Dis 1975;160:108–118.

Siefen G, Remschmidt H. Behandlungsergebnisse mit clozapin bei schizophrenen jugendlichen [Clozapine in the treatment of adolescents with schizophrenia: Treatment outcome]. Zeitschrift fur Kinder-und-Jugendpsychiatrie 1986; 14:245–257. (English translation by the Ralph McElroy Co., provided by the manufacturer.)

Simeon JG, Ferguson HB. Alprazolam effects in children with anxiety disorders. Can J Psychiatry 1987;32:570–574.

Simeon JG, Ferguson HB. Recent developments in the use of antidepressant and anxiolytic medications. Psychiatr Clin North Am 1985;8:893–907.

Sleator EK. Diagnosis. In: Sleator EK, Pelham WE Jr, eds. Attention deficit disorder. Dialogues in pediatric management, Vol. 1, No. 3. Norwalk, CT: Appleton-Century-Crofts, 1986:11–42.

Sleator EK, von Neumann A, Sprague RL. Hyperactive children: A continuous long-term placebo-controlled follow-up. JAMA 1974;229:316–317.

Smith TC, Wollman H. History and principles of anaesthesiology. In: Gilman AF, Goodman LS, Rall TW, Murad R, eds. Goodman and Gilman's the pharmacological basis of therapeutics. 7th ed. New York: Macmillan, 1985:260–275.

Sokol MS, Campbell M. Novel psychoactive agents in the

treatment of developmental disorders. In: Aman MG, Singh NN, eds. Psychopharmacology of the developmental disabilities. New York: Springer-Verlag, 1988, pp. 147–167.

Spitzer RL, Endicott J, Robins E. Research diagnostic criteria. Arch Gen Psychiatry 1978;35:773–782.

Sprague RL, Sleator EK. Methylphenidate in hyperkinetic children: Differences in dose effects on learning and social behavior. Science 1977;198:1274–1276.

Stanley B. An integration of ethical and clinical considerations in the use of placebos. Psychopharmacol Bull 1988;24:18–20.

Stores G. Antiepileptics (anticonvulsants). In: Werry JS, ed. Pediatric psychopharmacology: The use of behavior modifying drugs in children. New York: Brunner/Mazel, 1978:274–315.

Strayhorn JM, Rapp N, Donina W, Strain PS. Randomized trial of methylphenidate for an autistic child. J Am Acad Child Adolesc Psychiatry 1988;27:244–247.

Strober M, Freeman R, Rigali J. The pharmacotherapy of depressive illness in adolescents: I. An open label trial of imipramine. Psychopharmacol Bull 1990;26:80–84.

Sudden death in children treated with a tricyclic antidepressant. Med Letter 1990;32:53.

Swanson JM, Lerner M, Cantwell D. Blood levels and tolerance to stimulants in ADDH children. Clin Neuropharmacol 1986;9(suppl 4):523–525.

Teicher MH, Baldessarini RJ. Developmental pharmacodynamics. In: Popper C, ed. Psychiatric pharmacosciences of children and adolescents. Washington, DC: American Psychiatric Press, 1987:45–80.

United States Pharmacopeial Dispensing Information. Drug information for the health care professional. Rockville, MD: United States Pharmacopeial Convention, Inc., 1990.

Van Putten T, Marder SR. Behavioral toxicity of antipsychotic drugs. J Clin Psychiatry 1987;48(9)(suppl): 13–19.

Van Putten T, May PRA, Marder SR. Akathisia with haloperidol and thiothixene. Arch Gen Psychiatry 1984;41:1036–1039.

Varanka TM, Weller RA, Weller EB, Fristad MA. Lithium treatment of manic episodes with psychotic features in prepubertal children. Am J Psychiatry 1988;145:1557–1559.

Verglas, GDU, Banks SR, Guyer KE. Clinical effects of fenfluramine on children with autism: A review of the research. J Autism Dev Disord 1988;18:297–308.

Vetro A, Szentistvanyi I, Pallag L, Vargha M, Szilard J. Therapeutic experience with lithium in childhood aggressivity. Pharmacopsychiatry 1985;14:121–127.

Villeneuve A. The rabbit syndrome: A peculiar extrapyramidal reaction. Can Psychiatr Assoc J 1972;17:69–72.

Vincent J, Varley CK, Leger P. Effects of methylphenidate on early adolescent growth. Am J Psychiatry 1990;147:501–502.

Vitiello B, Behar D, Malone R, Delaney MA, Ryan PJ, Simpson GM. Pharmacokinetics of lithium carbonate in children. J Clin Psychopharmacol 1988;8:355–359.

Weiner JM, ed. Psychopharmacology in childhood and adolescence. New York: Basic Books, 1977.

Weiner JM, ed. Diagnosis and psychopharmacology of childhood and adolescent disorders. New York: John Wiley & Sons, 1985.

Weiner JM, Jaffe SL. Historical overview of childhood and adolescent psychopharmacoloy. In: Weiner JM, ed. Diagnosis and psychopharmacology of childhood and adolescent disorders. New York: John Wiley & Sons, 1985:3–50.

Weiner N. Norepinephrine, epinephrine, and the sympathomimetic amines. In: Gilman AG, Goodman LS, Gilman A, eds. Goodman and Gilman's the pharmacological basis of therapeutics. 6th ed. New York: Macmillan, 1980:138–175.

Weiss G, Hechtman LT. Hyperactive children grown up: Empirical findings and theoretical considerations. New York: Guilford Press, 1986.

Weizman A, Weitz R, Szekely GA, Tyano S, Belmaker RH. Combination of neuroleptic and stimulant treatment in attention deficit disorder with hyperactivity. J Am Acad Child Psychiatry 1984;23:295–298.

Weller EB, Weller RA, Fristad MA. Lithium dosage guide for prepubertal children: A preliminary report. J Am Acad Child Psychiatry 1986;25:92–95.

Weller EB, Weller RA, Fristad MA, Cantwell M, Tucker S. Saliva lithium monitoring in prepubertal children. J Am Acad Child Adolesc Psychiatry 1987;26:173–175.

Weller EB, Weller RA, Preskorn SH, Glotzbach R. Steady-state plasma imipramine levels in prepubertal depressed children. Am J Psychiatry 1982;139:506–508.

Wender PH. Attention deficit hyperactivity disorder. In: Howells JG, ed. Modern perspectives in clinical psychiatry. New York: Brunner/Mazel, 1988:149–169.

Wernicke JF. The side effect profile and safety of fluoxetine. J Clin Psychiatry 1985:46(3, sec. 2):59–67.

Werry JS, ed. Pediatric psychopharmacology: The use of behavior modifying drugs in children. New York: Brunner/Mazel, 1978.

Whalen CK, Henker B, Swanson JM, Granger D, Kliewer W, Spencer J. Natural social behaviors in hyperactive children: Dose effects of methylphenidate. J Consult Clin Psychol 1987;55:187–193.

White L, Tursky B, Schwartz GE, eds. Placebo: Theory, research, and mechanisms. New York: Guilford Press, 1985.

Williams DT, Mehl R, Yudofsky S, Adams D, Roseman B. The effect of propranolol on uncontrolled rage outbursts in children and adolescents with organic brain dysfunction. J Am Acad Child Psychiatry 1982;21:129–135.

Winsberg BG, Kupietz SS, Sverd J, Hungund BL, Young NL. Methylphenidate oral dose plasma concentrations and behavioral response in children. Psychopharmacology 1982;76:329–332.

Zametkin AJ, Rapoport JL. Noradrenergic hypothesis of attention deficit disorder with hyperactivity: A critical review. In: Meltzer HY, ed. Psychopharmacology: The third generation of progress. New York: Raven Press, 1987:837–842.

Zametkin A, Rapoport JL, Murphy DL, Linnoila M, Ismond D. Treatment of hyperactive children with monoamine oxidase inhibitors: I. Clinical Efficacy. Arch Gen Psychiatry 1985;42:962–966.

Zrull JP, Westman JC, Arthur B, Bell WA. A comparison of chlordiazepoxide, d-amphetamine, and placebo in the treatment of the hyperkinetic syndrome in children. Am J Psychiatry 1963;120:590–591.

Zrull JP, Westman JC, Arthur B, Rice DL. A comparison of diazepam, d-amphetamine, and placebo in the treatment of the hyperkinetic syndrome in children. Am J Psychiatry 1964;121:388–389.

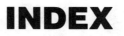

INDEX

Page numbers in *italics* denote figures; those followed by "t" denote tables.

Abnormal Involuntary Movement
  Scale, 28–29, 32, *34–37*
Abuse, drug (*see* Drugs, abuse)
Adjustment disorders, chlor-
  diazepoxide in, 163
α-Adrenergic antagonists (*see*
  Clonidine)
β-Adrenergic blockers (*see*
  Propranolol)
Adverse effects (*see* Untoward
  effects)
Aggressive conduct disorder (*see*
  Conduct disorder)
Agoraphobia, imipramine in, 119
Agranulocytosis
  with antipsychotic drugs, 82,
    91t–92t, 105–106
  with carbamazepine, 173
AIMS (Abnormal Involuntary Movement Scale), 28–29, 32, *34–37*
Akathisia, with antipsychotic drugs,
  18, 84–87, *88*
Akinesia, with antipsychotic drugs,
  84
Alcohol, interactions
  with antihistamines, 170
  with antipsychotic drugs, 81
  with phenytoin, 177
  with propranolol, 181
  with tricyclic antidepressants, 111
Alprazolam
  dosage, 162t
  in avoidance disorder, 167
  in cancer patients, 166
  in night terrors, 166
  in separation anxiety disorder, 167
American Psychiatric Association
  diagnostic nomenclature,
    7–10
Amitriptyline, 125
Amphetamines (*see also*
  Dextroamphetamine)
  dyskinesia with, 90
  historical perspective, 53
  in attention deficit hyperactivity
    disorder, 61–62
  intelligence, effection, 53
Anafranil (*see* Clomipramine)

Anticholinergic drugs, interactions
  with antipsychotic drugs, 81,
    85–86
Anticholinergic effects
  with antipsychotics, 81, 91t
  with diphenhydramine, 172
  with tricyclic antidepressants,
    110, 112
Antidepressants
  amitriptyline, 125
  bupropion hydrochloride,
    140–142
  clomipramine (*see* Clomipramine)
  desipramine (*see* Desipramine)
  fluoxetine, 137–139
  imipramine (*see* Imipramine)
  monoamine oxidase inhibitors (*see*
    Monoamine oxidase
    inhibitors)
  nortriptyline, 38, 120–124, 124t
  tricyclic (*see* Tricyclic
    antidepressants)
Antiepileptic drugs, 173–178
  carbamazepine, 145, 173–177
  dyskinesia with, 90
  phenytoin, 65, 174, 177–178, 181
Antihistamines, 170–173
  contraindications, 170
  diphenhydramine, 83, 86,
    171–172
  dosage, 171–173
  dyskinesia with, 90
  hydroxyzine, 170, 172–173
  indications, 170
  interactions, 170
    with antipsychotic drugs, 81
    with stimulants, 65
Antipsychotic drugs, 78–107, *90*,
    94t–95t (*see also specific
    drug*)
  agranulocytosis with, 82, 91t–92t,
    105–106
  akathisia with, 84–87
  antiparkinsonian agents with,
    85–87
  chlorprothixene, 94t, 100
  clozapine, 94t, 105–107
  cognitive impairment with, 82

Antipsychotic drugs *continued*
contraindications, 81
dosage, 90, 94t-95t
drug holiday and, 42–43
dystonic reactions to, 83, 85–87
extrapyramidal syndromes with,
82–83, 94t-95t
fluphenazine, 95t, 97, 101–102
haloperidol (*see* Haloperidol)
indications, 78–80
interactions, 81–82
with antihistamines, 170
with lithium, 144–145
with tricyclic antidepressants,
111
loxapine succinate, 94t, 100–101
malignant neuroleptic syndrome
with, 87
metabolism, 78, 80–81
parkinsonism with, 83–87
perioral tremor with, 90
pharmacokinetics, 80–81
pimozide, 95t, 97, 102–105
rabbit syndrome with, 90
seizure threshold and, 28
tardive dyskinesia with, 87–90
thiothixene, 95t, 99–100
trifluoperazine, 95t, 96
untoward effects, 82–90, 91t-92t
during administration, 83–87
late-appearing, 87–90
with stimulants, 80
withdrawal from, 50
dyskinesia in, 89
Anxiety
antipsychotic drugs in, 96
anxiolytics in (*see also* Benzodiazepines)
buspirone, 167–169
interactions with anti-
histamines, 170
carbamazepine in, 176
diphenhydramine in, 171
hydroxyzine in, 172
overanxious disorder
alprazolam in, 167
buspirone in, 169
diphenhydramine in, 171
propranolol in, 180
separation (*see* Separation anxiety
disorder)
Anxiolytics (*see under* Anxiety;
Benzodiazepines)
Artane (trihexyphenidyl), in
akathisia, 85

Atarax (*see* Hydroxyzine)
Ativan (lorazepam), dosage, 162t
Attention deficit hyperactivity
disorder
antidepressants in
bupropion, 141–142
clomipramine, 132–133
desipramine, 126–129
imipramine, 118–119
monoamine oxidase inhibitors,
136–137
antipsychotic drugs in, 79–80
haloperidol, 96
propericiazine, 80
thioridazine, 93
catecholamine function and,
12–13
clonidine in, 185–187
definition, 10
lithium in, 156
propranolol in, 182
stimulants in
amphetamines, 61–62
caffeine, 77
dextroamphetamine, 62–63,
66–67, 73–74
fenfluramine, 76–77
magnesium pemoline, 65, 75–76
methylphenidate, 16, 61–62,
66–73, 186–187
treatment plan development for,
15–16
vs. Tourette's disorder, 68
with Tourette's disorder, 128–129
Atypical pervasive developmental
disorders
fluphenazine in, 102
haloperidol in, 98–99
Autistic disorder (see also pervasive
developmental disorders)
antihistamines in, 171
antipsychotic drugs in, 78, 98
buspirone in, 169
diphenhydramine in, 171
fenfluramine in, 77
haloperidol in, 98
methylphenidate in, 72–73
naltrexone in, 179–180
propranolol in, 182
Autonomic effects, with antipsychotic drugs, 94t-95t
Avoidance disorder, alprazolam in,
167
Azaspirodecamediones, as anxiolytic, 167–169

Barbiturates
  interactions
    with antihistamines, 170
    with antipsychotic drugs, 81
    with tricyclic antidepressants, 111
  untoward effects, 189–190
Baseline assessment (see Premedication workup)
Behavior, premedication assessment, 28–29, *30–31*, 32, *34–37*
Behavior disorders (see also Conduct disorder)
  carbamazepine in, 175–177
  phenytoin in, 177–178
Behavioral toxicity, 41
Benadryl (see Diphenhydramine)
Benzedrine (see Amphetamines)
Benzodiazepines, 157–167
  abuse, 157
  contraindications, 160
  dosage, 161, 162t
  dyskinesia with, 90
  in antipsychotic drug reaction, 85
  indications, 157–161, 162t
  interactions, 160
    with antipsychotic drugs, 81
    with phenytoin, 177
    with stimulants, 65
    with tricyclic antidepressants, 111
  types, 162t
  untoward effects, 161
Benztropine, in antipsychotic drug reaction, 83, 86
Bipolar disorder
  carbamazepine in, 174
  lithium therapy in (see Lithium carbonate)
  misdiagnosis, drug response in, 8–9
Blood dyscrasia
  with clomipramine, 131
  with tricyclic antidepressants, 112
Bupropion hydrochloride
  contraindications, 140
  dosage, 140
  in attention deficit hyperactivity disorder, 141–142
  indications, 140
  interactions, 140–141
  untoward effects, 141
Buspirone hydrochloride (BuSpar), as anxiolytic, 167–169

Caffeine, in attention deficit hyperactivity disorder, 77
Calcium metabolism, in lithium therapy, 150–151
Cancer patients, anxiety in, alprazolam in, 166
CAPTQ (Conners Parent-Teacher Questionnaire), 29, *30–31*, 32
Carbamazepine
  contraindications, 174
  in bipolar disorder, 174
  indications, 174–177
  interactions, 174
    with lithium, 145
    with phenytoin, 177
  untoward effects, 173, 176
Cardiac arrhythmia
  with clozapine, 106
  with pimozide, 103
Cardiotoxicity
  with desipramine, 127–128
  with imipramine, 113
  with lithium, 28, 150
  with tricyclic antidepressants, 27, 111–112
Caretaker, relationship to, 15–20
Catapres (see Clonidine)
Catecholamine function, in children vs. adults, 12–13
Central nervous system toxicity, with tricyclic antidepressants, 112
Chlorazepate, dosage, 162t
Chlordiazepoxide
  dosage, 162t
  in behavior disorders, 162–164
  untoward effects, 163
Chlorpromazine
  dosage, 92–93, 94t
  generic vs. trade preparation, 38
  in mental retardation, 79
  indications, 92
  interaction with propranolol, 181
  pharmacokinetics, 13, 80–81
  serum monitoring, 48
  untoward effects, 82, 91t–92t
Chlorprothixene, 94t, 100
Cholinergic overdrive phenomenon, in antidepressant withdrawal, 110
Choreoathetoid movement
  in tardive dyskinesia, 88
  with magnesium pemoline, 76
Cibalith-S (lithium citrate syrup), 151–152

Clinical record, medicolegal aspects, 24–25
Clomipramine
  dosage, 130
    children vs. adults, 13
  in attention deficit hyperactivity disorder, 126, 132–133
  in enuresis, 133
  in obsessive-compulsive disorder, 129, 131–132
  in separation anxiety disorder, 134
  indications, 108, 130
  mechanism of action, 129–130
  pharmacokinetics, 13, 130–131
  serum monitoring, 48
  untoward effects, 131
  withdrawal from, 130
Clonazepam, in antipsychotic drug reaction, 85
Clonidine, 183–189
  contraindications, 184
  dosage, 184–185
  in antipsychotic drug reaction, 85
  in attention deficit hyperactivity disorder, 185–187
  in Tourette's disorder, 188–189
  indications, 184
  interactions, 184
  mechanism of action, 183–184
  pharmacokinetics, 184
  transdermal patch, 185
  untoward effects, 186, 189
  withdrawal from, 185
Clorgyline
  in attention deficit hyperactivity disorder, 136
  in depression, 134
Clozapine (Clozaril)
  agranulocytosis with, 105–106
  dosage, 94t, 105
  in schizophrenia, 106–107
  indications, 105
  untoward effects, 105–106
Cocaine, interactions with stimulants, 65
Cogentin (benztropine), 83, 86
Cognitive factors, in psychopharmacotherapy, 14–15
Cognitive impairment, with antipsychotic drugs, 82
Compliance, with treatment plan, 17–19
Conduct disorder
  chlordiazepoxide in, 163–164
  severely aggressive
    antipsychotics in, 79

    chlorpromazine, 92–93
    haloperidol, 96–97, 99, 155
    thioridazine, 93
  carbamazepine in, 176
  lithium in, 79, 155–156
  methylphenidate in, 178
  phenytoin in, 178
  propranolol in, 182–183
Conners rating instruments, 29, 30–31, 32
CPQ (Conners Parent Questionnaire), 29, 32
CTQ (Conners Teacher Questionnaire), 29, 32
Cylert (see Magnesium pemoline)

Dalmane (flurazepam), dosage, 162t
L-Deprenyl
  in attention deficit hyperactivity disorder, 136–137
  in depression, 134
Depression, treatment (see Antidepressants)
Desipramine
  dosage, 126–129
  in attention deficit hyperactivity disorder, 126–129
  in enuresis, 126
  in tics, 126–129
  indications, 126
  pharmacokinetics, 109
  serum monitoring, 48
  sudden death with, 111–112
  untoward effects, 127–129
Desmethylclomipramine, as clomipramine metabolite, 129–131
Developmental disorders, pervasive
  dextroamphetamine in, 74
  fluphenazine in, 102
  haloperidol in, 98–99
Developmental issues, 12–14
Developmental neurotoxicity, of drugs, 13–14
Dexedrine (see Dextroamphetamine)
Dextroamphetamine
  dosage, 74
  in attention deficit hyperactivity disorder, 62–63, 66–67, 73–74, 136
  in pervasive developmental disorders, 74
  in sleep disorders, 71
  indications, 73
  pharmacokinetics, 64t

rebound effects, 66
untoward effects, 65–66
Diagnosis
    changing criteria, 9–10
    incorrect, drug response in, 8–9
    medicolegal aspects, 21–22
    nomenclature problems, 7–10
    target symptoms and, 11–12
*Diagnostic and Statistical Manual of
    Mental Disorders*, 7–8, 10
Diazepam
    dosage, 162t
    in enuresis, 165–166
    in schizophrenia, 165
    in sleep disorders, 166
    interaction with fluoxetine, 138
Dilantin (*see* Phenytoin)
Diphenhydramine
    dosage, 171–172
    in antipsychotic drug reactions,
        83, 86
    indications, 171
    interactions, 170
    untoward effects, 172
Diphenylhydantoin (*see* Phenytoin)
Documentation, in clinical record,
    medicolegal aspects, 24–25
L-Dopa, dyskinesia with, 90
Dosage (*see also specific drug*)
    children vs. adults, 12–14
    discontinuation, 25
    increases, 43–44, 51
    initial, 40–41
    optimal, 44–45
    regulation, 40–45
    scheduling, 41–42
    tapering down, 25, 49–50
    titration, 44
Drugs
    abuse
        benzodiazepines, 157
        screening for, 40
        stimulants, 65, 68
    disposition (*see* Pharmacokinetics)
    dosage (*see* Dosage; *specific drug*)
    effectiveness in multiple disor-
        ders, 8
    generic, 33, 38
    holiday from, 42–43
    interactions, 39–40 (*see also spe-
        cific drug*)
        medicolegal aspects, 21–22
    investigational uses, 39
    manufacturer's labeling, deviating
        from, 5, 24, 58
    mechanisms of action, 8

monitoring serum levels (*see*
    Monitoring)
non-approved use, 39
    medicolegal aspects, 24
nonstandard treatment with, 24, 39
refractoriness to, 8
response to
    evaluation, in absence of effec-
        tive communication, 14–15
    in incorrect diagnosis, 8–9
    individual variations, 8
    patient description, 19
selection
    importance of correct diagnosis,
        7–10
    initial, 33
    target symptoms and, 11–12
standard treatment with, 39
trade preparations vs. generic, 33,
    38
Dyskinesia
    acute, as drug reaction, 90
    tardive (*see* Tardive dyskinesia)
Dystonia, with antipsychotic drugs,
    83, 85–88

Elavil (amitriptyline), 125
Electrocardiography
    in tricyclic therapy, 22, 27, 111,
        114, 115, 121
    in lithium therapy, 28, 150
    in premedication workup, 27–28
Electroencephalography
    in lithium therapy, 28, 151
    in premedication workup, 28, 151
Emergency, involuntary treatment
    in, 23
Encopresis, lithium in, 156
Endep (amitriptyline), 125
Enuresis
    amphetamines in, 53
    antidepressants in, 109
    clomipramine, 133
    desipramine, 126
    imipramine, 113–114
    carbamazepine in, 176
    diazepam in, 165–166
    with lithium therapy, 148
Epilepsy, drugs for, in psychiatric
    disorders, 173–178
Eskalith (*see* Lithium carbonate)
Experiential factors, in psychophar-
    macotherapy, 14–15
Extrapyramidal syndromes, with
    antipsychotic drugs, 82–83
    treatment, 86

Family, relationship to, 15–20
  medicolegal aspects, 20–21
Fenfluramine
  in attention deficit hyperactivity
    disorder, 76–77
  in autistic disorder, 77
  indications, 77
Fluoxetine
  contraindications, 138
  dosage, 137
  in major depressive disorder, 139
  in obsessive-compulsive disorder,
    139
  in Tourette's disorder, 139
  indications, 137
  interactions, 138
  mechanism of action, 137
  pharmacokinetics, 138
  untoward effects, 138–139
Fluphenazine
  dosage, 95t, 101–102
  in atypical pervasive developmen-
    tal disorders, 102
  indications, 101
Flurazepam, dosage, 162t
Food and Drug Administration
  approved drug use, deviation
    from, 5–6, 24, 58
  generic drug ratings, 33, 38

Generic drugs, 33, 38
Growth disturbances, in stimulant
  use, 66
Guardian, relationship to, 15–20

Halcion (triazolam)
  dosage, 162t
  in sleep onset insomnia, 159
Haldol (see Haloperidol)
Haloperidol
  dosage, 95t, 97
  drug holiday and, 43
  in aggressive conduct disorder,
    96–97, 99, 155
  in attention deficit hyperactivity
    disorder, 96
  in atypical pervasive developmen-
    tal disorders, 98–99
  in autistic disorder, 98
  in mental retardation, 79
  in Tourette's disorder, 96–97
  indications, 96, 98–99
  interaction with carbamazepine,
    174
  pharmacokinetics, 97
  serum monitoring, 47, 48

  untoward effects, 45, 98, 99, 100
Heart block, with tricyclic anti-
  depressants, 111–112
Holiday, from drug regimen, 42–43
Hospitalization
  for premedication observation, 29
  medicolegal aspects, 21
Hydroxyzine, 172–173
  interactions, 170
Hyperactivity (see also Attention
    deficit hyperactivity disorder)
  as target symptom, 11
Hyperkinesis, carbamazepine-
    induced, 176
Hypertensive crisis, in monoamine
    oxidase inhibitor therapy,
    135–136
Hypnotics
  interactions
    with antihistamines, 170
    with antipsychotic drugs, 81
  untoward effects, 189–190
Hypocalciuria, with lithium,
    150–151
Hypotension, orthostatic, with
    clozapine, 106–107

Imipramine
  baseline studies for, 115
  dosage, 112–114, 119
  in attention deficit hyperactivity
    disorder, 118–119
  in enuresis, 113–114
  in major depressive disorder
    adolescent, 117–118
    prepubertal, 115–117
  in night terrors, 120
  in separation anxiety disorder, 119
  in somnambulism, 120
  indications, 108, 113
  pharmacokinetics, 13, 109, 115–116
  serum monitoring, 48, 109, 115–
    118
  sudden death from, 111
  untoward effects, 113, 116–117
Inderal (propranolol), 85, 180–182
Informed consent, medicolegal
    aspects, 22–23
Insomnia
  antihistamines in
    diphenhydramine, 171
    hydroxyzine, 172
  benzodiazepines in, 159
  methylphenidate-induced, 70–71
Intelligence, amphetamines effect
    on, 53

Interactions, drugs (see under Drugs)
Intermittent explosive disorder, propranolol in, 182
Investigational use of drugs, 39 (see also specific drug)
Involuntary treatment, medicolegal aspects, 23
Isocarboxazid, in depression, 134

Kidney function tests
in lithium therapy, 149–150
premedication, 27

Laboratory tests
in drug serum level monitoring, 46–48
in lithium therapy, 146, 149–153
in premedication workup, 26–27, 149–153
Legal aspects (see Medicolegal aspects)
Leukocytosis, with lithium, 149
Libido changes, with tricyclic antidepressants, 112
Librium (chlordiazepoxide), 162–164, 162t
Lithane (see Lithium carbonate)
Lithium carbonate, 143–156
cardiotoxicity, 28
contraindications, 144
dosage, 12, 152–153
in behavioral disorders, 154–155
in children under 12, 153–154, 154t
in mood disorders, 154–155
in patients with lithium-responding parents, 154–155
dyskinesia with, 90
in aggressive conduct disorder, 79, 155–156
in attention deficit hyperactivity disorder, 156
in major depressive disorder, 118
in patients with lithium-responding parents, 154–155
indications, 11, 143, 151–152
interactions, 144–145
with antipsychotic drugs, 81
with carbamazepine, 174
laboratory testing, 146, 149–153
monitoring, 146, 151–153
pharmacokinetics, 47, 143–144
premedication workup, 27, 28, 149–151
prophylactic use, 153

seizure threshold and, 28
teratogenic effects, 144, 149
therapeutic index, 145–146
toxicity, 28, 145–147
untoward effects, 147–148, 152
Lithium citrate syrup, 151–152
Lithobid (see Lithium carbonate)
Lorazepam, dosage, 162t
Loxapine (Loxitane)
dosage, 94t, 101
indications, 100

Magnesium pemoline
dosage, 75
in attention deficit hyperactivity disorder, 65, 75–76
indications, 75
pharmacokinetics, 13, 64t, 75
tics and, 67
Major depressive disorder (see also Antidepressants)
fluoxetine in, 139
imipramine in
adolescent, 117–118
prepubertal, 115–117
lithium prophylaxis in, 153
monoamine oxidase inhibitors in, 136
nortriptyline in
adolescent, 122–124, 124t
prepubertal, 121–124, 124t
Major tranquilizers (see Antipsychotic drugs)
Malpractice (see also, medicolegal aspects), 21
Mania, carbamazepine-induced, 176
Manic-depressive illness, drugs for (see Antipsychotic drugs; Lithium carbonate)
Marplan (isocarboxazid), in depression, 143
Maturational issues, 12–14
Medicolegal aspects, 20–25
clinical record, 24–25
diagnostic accuracy, 21–22
drug administration decisions, 23
drug interactions, 21–22
drug manufacturer label recommendations, 24
family relationship, 20–21
Food and Drug Administration-approved indications, 24
informed consent, 22–23
involuntary treatment, 23
premedication workup, 21–22
suicide, 21, 23

Mellaril (*see* Thioridazine)
Mental retardation
  antipsychotics in, 79
  haloperidol in, 79
  lithium in, 153
  propranolol in, 182
  stimulants in, 57, 63
  controversy on, 9–10
Mesoridazine, dosage, 94t
Methylphenidate
  dosage, 17, 69–72
  dyskinesia with, 90
  in aggressive conduct disorder,
      178
  in attention deficit hyperactivity
      disorder, 16, 56, 61–62,
      66–73, 126, 186–187
  in autistic disorder, 72–73
  indications, 69
  interaction with phenytoin, 177
  pharmacokinetics, 64t, 69–70
  rebound effects, 66
  serum monitoring, 48
  sustained-release, 70
  tics caused by, 67
  tolerance to, 72
  untoward effects, 65–66, 70–72
  withdrawal from, 49–51
Minimal brain dysfunction
  amphetamines in, 62
  definition, 9–10
  in Tourette's disorder, 68
  phenytoin in, 178
Molindone (Moban)
  dosage, 95t
  interaction with phenytoin, 177
Monitoring, drug serum levels,
      46–48
  imipramine, 48, 109, 115–118
  lithium, 146, 151–153
  nortriptyline, 122–124
Monoamine oxidase inhibitors,
      134–139
  contraindications, 135
  dyskinesia with, 90
  fluoxetine, 137–139
  in adolescent depression, 136
  in attention deficit hyperactivity
      disorder, 136–137
  indications, 134
  interactions, 135–136
    with antihistamines, 170
    with antipsychotic drugs, 81–82
    with stimulants, 65
    with tricyclic antidepressants,
        110–111

special considerations, 135
types, 134
untoward effects, 136
Moodiness, carbamazepine in, 175
Motor restlessness, with antipsy-
      chotic drugs, 84–87
Motor tic disorder, antipsychotic
      drugs in, 79
Movement
  choreoathetoid
    in tardive dyskinesia, 88
    with magnesium pemoline, 76
  involuntary, rating scales for,
      28–29, 32, 34–37
Muscular hypotonicity, with anti-
      psychotic drugs, 83

Naltrexone, 179–180
Narcotics, interactions with anti-
      histamines, 170
Nardil (phenelzine sulfate), in
      depression, 134, 136
Navane (thiothixene), 95t, 99–100
Neuroleptic malignant syndrome, 87
Neuroleptics (*see* Antipsychotic
      drugs)
Neurotoxicity, developmental, of
      drugs, 13–14
Night terrors
  alprazolam in, 166
  benzodiazepines in, 158–159, 166
  carbamazepine in, 175–176
  diazepam in, 166
  imipramine in, 120
Norfluoxetine, as fluoxetine metabo-
      lite, 138
Norpramine (*see* Desipramine)
Nortriptyline
  dosage, 120–124, 124t
  generic vs. trade preparation, 38
  in major depressive disorder
    adolescent, 122–124, 124t
    dosage, 123–124, 124t
    prepubertal, 121–124, 124t
  indications, 120
  monitoring serum levels, 122–124
  withdrawal from, 124

Obsessive-compulsive disorder
  antidepressants in, fluoxetine, 139
  clomipramine, 129, 131–132
Oculogyric crisis, with antipsychotic
      drugs, 83
Opiate antagonists, 178–180
Opiates, interactions with anti-
      psychotic drugs, 81

Opisthotonos, with antipsychotic
drugs, 83
Orap (see Pimozide)
Organic brain dysfunction, pro-
pranolol in, 181–182
Orthostatic hypotension, with
clozapine, 106–107
Overanxious disorder (see Anxiety)
Oxazepam, dosage, 162t

Pamelor (see Nortriptyline)
Panic disorder, imipramine in, 119
Parkinsonism, with antipsychotic
drugs, 83–87
Parnate (tranylcypromine sulfate),
134, 136
Pavor nocturnus (see Night terrors)
Pemoline (see Magnesium pemoline)
Penfluridol, in Tourette's disorder,
97
Perioral tremor, with antipsychotic
drugs, 90
Permitil (see Fluphenazine)
Perphenazine, dosage, 95t
Personality disorder, chlordiazepoxide in, 164
Pertofrane (see Desipramine)
Pervasive developmental disorders
see also autistic disorder
dextroamphetamine in, 74
fluphenazine in, 102
haloperidol in, 98–99
Pharmacokinetics (see also specific
drug)
acute vs. chronic, 13
children vs. adults, 12–14
dosage scheduling and, 41–42
drug serum level monitoring and,
46–48
interindividual variations, 37
Phenelzine sulfate, in depression,
134, 136
Phenobarbital
interactions
with carbamazepine, 174
with stimulants, 65
untoward effects, 189–190
Phenobarbitone, interaction with
propranolol, 181
Phenothiazines, interactions with
phenytoin, 177
Phenytoin, 177–178
interactions
with carbamazepine, 174
with propranolol, 181
with stimulants, 65

Physical examination, in premedication workup, 26
Physiological factors, in psychopharmacotherapy, 12–14
Pimozide
contraindications, 103
dosage, 95t, 102
in Tourette's disorder, 97,
103–104
indications, 102
pharmacokinetics, 103
untoward effects, 103
Placebos, 54–56
Polydipsia, with lithium, 148
Polypharmacy, 23
Polyuria, with lithium, 148
Pondimin (fenfluramine), 76–77
Posttraumatic stress disorder, propranolol in, 183
Pregnancy, teratogenic drugs in, 26
lithium, 144, 149
Premedication workup, 25–33
behavioral assessment, 28–29,
30–31, 32, 34–37
components, 25–26
electrocardiography in, 27–28, 150
electroencephalography in, 28, 151
laboratory tests in, 26–27
lithium therapy, 149–153
medicolegal aspects, 21–22
physical examination in, 26
Primidone, interaction with carbamazepine, 174
Prolixin (see Fluphenazine)
Propericiazine, in attention deficit
hyperactivity disorder, 80
Propranolol
contraindications, 181
in antipsychotic drug reaction, 85
indications, 180–182
interactions, 181
mechanism of action, 180
untoward effects, 181
Prozac (fluoxetine), 137–139
Pseudoparkinsonism, with antipsychotic drugs, 83–87
Psychological factors, in psychopharmacotherapy, 14–15
Psychopharmacotherapy, historical
perspective, 53–54
Psychosis, drug-induced
in incorrect diagnosis, 9
with tricyclic antidepressants, 112

Rabbit syndrome, with antipsychotic
drugs, 90

Rage, uncontrolled, propranolol in, 182
Rating scales, for behavioral assessment, 28–29, *30–31*, 32, *34–37*
Recordkeeping, medicolegal aspects, 24–25
Research studies
  behavioral rating scales in, 28–29, *30–31*, 32, *34–37*
  evaluation, 56–57
  placebos in, 54–56
Restlessness, with antipsychotic drugs, 84–87
Restoril (temazepam), dosage, 162t
Rifampin, interaction with propranolol, 181
Ritalin (*see* Methylphenidate)

Saliva test, for lithium monitoring, 146
Schizophrenia
  antihistamines in, 171
  antipsychotic drugs in, 78
    clozapine, 105–107
    loxapine, 101
    thiothixene, 99–100
  as incorrect diagnosis, drug response in, 8–9
  chlordiazepoxide in, 164
  diazepam in, 165
  diphenhydramine in, 171
  stimulant-induced, 68
  tricyclic antidepressants contraindicated in, 111
School phobia (*see* Separation anxiety disorder)
Sedation
  with antipsychotic drugs, 94t-95t
  with diphenhydramine, 172
Sedatives, interactions with antipsychotic drugs, 81
Seizures
  dextroamphetamine and, 74
  methylphenidate and, 71–72
  with antipsychotics, 28
  with bupropion, 140–141
  with clomipramine, 131
  with clozapine, 106
  with imipramine, 113
  with tricyclic antidepressants, 28, 110, 113
Semap (penfluridol), 97
Separation anxiety disorder (school phobia)
  alprazolam in, 167

antidepressants in
  clomipramine, 134
  imipramine, 119
buspirone in, 169
chlordiazepoxide in, 163–164
Serax (oxazepam), dosage, 162t
Serentil (mesoridazine), dosage, 94t
Side effects (*see* Untoward effects)
Sleep disorders
  benzodiazepines in, 158–159, 161, 166
  carbamazepine in, 175–176
  chlordiazepoxide in, 162
  dextroamphetamine in, 71
  diazepam in, 166
  diphenhydramine in, 171
  hydroxyzine in, 172
  imipramine in, 120
  with methylphenidate, 70–71
Sleep terror disorder (*see* Night terrors)
Sleepwalking (somnambulism)
  benzodiazepines in, 158–159
  diazepam in, 166
  imipramine in, 120
Smoking, interactions with tricyclic antidepressants, 111
Sodium levels, in lithium therapy, 147
Somnambulism (*see* Sleepwalking)
Spasms, muscular, with antipsychotic drugs, 83
Stelazine (trifluoperazine), 95t, 96
Stereotypy
  in autistic disorder, haloperidol and, 98
  stimulant-induced, 67
Stimulants, 61–77
  abuse, 65, 68
  caffeine, 77
  contraindications, 63, 65
  dextroamphetamine (*see* Dextroamphetamine)
  drug holiday and, 42
  fenfluramine, 76–77
  in mental retardation, 57
    controversy on, 9–10
  indications, 61–63
  interactions, 65
  magnesium pemoline (*see* Magnesium pemoline)
  methylphenidate (*see* Methylphenidate)
  pharmacokinetics, 63, 64t
  psychosis caused by, in unrecognized schizophrenia, 9

rebound effects, 66
tics and, 67–69
tolerance to, 62–63
Tourette's disorder and, 67–69
untoward effects, 63, 65–66
with antipsychotic drugs, 80
Sudden death, with tricyclic antidepressants, 111–112
Suicide, medicolegal aspects, 21, 23
Sympathomimetic drugs (see also
Stimulants)
interactions, with monoamine oxidase inhibitors, 135–136
Symptoms
target, diagnosis and, 11–12
withdrawal (see Withdrawal)

Taractan (chlorprothixene), 94t, 100
Tardive akathisia, with antipsychotic
drugs, 88
Tardive dyskinesia
definition, 87–88
prevalence, 89
symptoms, 88–89
treatment, 88–89
with antipsychotics, 42–43, 87–90
with haloperidol, 98
withdrawal-emergent, 89
Tardive dystonia, with antipsychotic
drugs, 88
Target symptoms, diagnosis and,
11–12
Tegretol (see Carbamazepine)
Temazepam, dosage, 162t
Temper tantrums, phenytoin in, 178
Teratogenesis, drugs in, 26
lithium carbonate, 144, 149
Tetrabenzine, in tardive dyskinesia,
88–89
Theophylline, interaction with carbamazepine, 174
Thioridazine
dosage, 93, 94t
in mental retardation, 79
indications, 93
Thiothixene
dosage, 95t, 99
in schizophrenia, 99–100
indications, 99
Thorazine (see Chlorpromazine)
Thyroid function, premedication
evaluation, 27
lithium therapy and, 144, 150
Tics
antipsychotic drugs in, 96–97
desipramine in, 126–129

stimulant effect on, 67–69
Time, child's concept, 14–15
Titration, dosage, 44
Tofranil (see Imipramine)
Torticollis, with antipsychotic drugs,
83
Tourette's disorder
antipsychotic drugs in, 79
haloperidol, 96–97
pimozide, 103–105
clonidine in, 188–189
fluoxetine in, 139
stimulant effect on, 67–69
vs. early attention deficit hyperactivity disorder, 68
with attention deficit hyperactivity disorder, 128–129
Tranquilizers, major (see Antipsychotic drugs)
Tranxene (chlorazepate), dosage,
162t
Tranylcypromine sulfate
in attention deficit hyperactivity
disorder, 136
in depression, 134, 136
Treatment plan, development, 15–17
Tremor, perioral, with antipsychotic
drugs, 90
Trexan (naltrexone), 179–180
Triazolam, dosage, 162t
Tricyclic antidepressants, 108–134
(see also specific drug)
amitriptyline, 125
cardiotoxicity, 27
clomipramine (see Clomipramine)
contraindications, 110–111
desipramine, 48, 109, 112,
126–129
dyskinesia with, 90
imipramine (see Imipramine)
indications, 108–109
interactions, 110–111
with antipsychotic drugs,
81–82, 111
with clonidine, 184
with monoamine oxidase inhibitors, 135
with phenytoin, 177
with stimulants, 65
nortriptyline, 38, 120–124, 124t
pharmacokinetics, 109, 110t
prophylactic use, 109
seizure threshold and, 28
serum monitoring, 48
sudden death, 111–112
toxicity, 109, 110t

Tricyclic antidepressants *continued*
  untoward effects, 111–112
  withdrawal from, 50, 109–110
Trifluoperazine, 95t, 96
Trihexyphenidyl, in akathisia, 85
Trilafon (perphenazine), dosage, 95t
Tyramine reaction, in monoamine
        oxidase inhibitor therapy, 135

Untoward effects, 45–46 *(see also
        specific drug)*
  behavioral toxicity, 41
  compliance and, 18
  description to patient, 19–20
  from drug withdrawal, 49–51
  sudden death, 111–112
  management, 46
  vs. withdrawal, 17
  withdrawl syndromes, 49–50

Valium (*see* Diazepam)
Valproic acid, interaction with phe-
        nytoin, 177

Vistaril (hydroxyzine), 170, 172–173
Vocal tic disorder, antipsychotic
        drugs in, 79

Wellbutrin (bupropion hydro-
        chloride), 140–142
Withdrawal
  compliance problems and, 17
  from antidepressants, 109–110
  from antipsychotic drugs, dyski-
        nesia in, 89
  from clomipramine, 130
  from clonidine, 185
  from nortriptyline, 124
  periodic, 42, 49
  symptoms, 49–50
  sundromes, 49–50
  untoward effects in, 49–51
  vs. untoward effects, 17

Xanax (alprazolam), 162t, 166–167